TWO ASPIRIN – FIRST DOSE

by John N. Withers, MD, FACS

IPO PUBLISHING COMPANY
P.O. Box 1490
Kahului, Maui, Hawaii 96732

International Standard Book Number: 0-9624722-0-4

Library of Congress Catalog Card Number: 89-81186

Withers, MD, FACS, John N.

Two Aspirin – First Dose

A collection of fifty articles covers a wide variety of medical concerns. Articles provide information and advice about medical problems in a style that is interesting and easy to understand by a non-medically oriented audience. Index. 96 pages.

Published and Distributed by   Ipo Publishing Company
P.O. Box 1490
Kahului, Maui, Hawaii, USA 96732

I dedicate this book to my partner in life . . . my wife, Carole.

DISCLAIMER

The purpose of this book is to educate and entertain the reader regarding certain medical topics which may have a bearing on his/her health. This book is not to be used as a "self-diagnosis" or a "self-treatment" book. It is not to replace visits to the appropriate physicians when they are indicated. The reader may worsen his condition if unnecessary delay occurs. The author, any co-writers, editors and publishers of this book shall have neither liability nor responsibility to any person or entity with respect to any loss or damage caused or alleged to be caused directly or indirectly by the information contained in this book.

TABLE OF CONTENTS

INTRODUCTION

People learn about medical care in many ways. The first is probably from their mothers."Johnny, take your vitamin so that you will grow tall and strong." Later, we tend to believe our peers, although they may know less that we know. Finally, when we mature to an age when we start worrying about our health, we begin reading every medical article we find. Unfortunately, most articles are rather dry and technical, and most people lose interest rather quickly. Of course the family physician is the best source of medical advice. Even though an appointment costs money, it is well worth the expense when a person is sick.

Newspaper and magazine articles are excellent sources of occasional medical information. More complete, categorized information can be found in a number of "home diagnosis" books, but these are hardly "evening-time" reading material. An excellent example is *The American Medical Association Family Medical Guide*, published by Random House. Over 800 pages, this reference deals with medical emergencies, self-diagnosis, healthy life styles, and many more subjects. It is crossed-referenced very well so that the information can be obtained easily. Although an excellent book, it is not one you would take with you for "light reading" on your flight from Honolulu to San Francisco.

For the past eight years I have authored the "Two Aspirin" column in *The Maui News*. The articles make medical learning both educational and enjoyable for the reader. This book is a collection of 50 articles from that column.

Just as continuing medical education is a life-long process for the physician, it must also be for the reader. After four years of medical school, a year of internship and four years of a surgical residency, I still learn something new every day. The field of medicine is advancing so rapidly that 50% of today's medical knowledge will be outdated in ten years! So if the reader learns 50 new medical ideas in a couple evenings of reading **Two Aspirin, First Dose**, I will consider that my time has been well spent in writing the book.

While preparing the articles for *The Maui News*, I would frequently forget that most readers do not have a large medical vocabulary. Not everyone knows that the sternocleidomastoid muscle is simply one of the neck muscles. This is when I would rely on my wife, Carole, who would proofread all the columns. Her questions, "What do you mean by this?" or "Can't you say it another way?", made the articles more readable and enjoyable.

I want to thank Victor C. Pellegrino, author and teacher of writing and literature at Maui Community College, for his help in editing and guidance in publishing. Rose Evans, my office medical secretary, deserves a great deal of credit for her encouragement and help in editing the articles during the two years of the book's development.

The medical advice offered in the book is not intended to replace the advice of a doctor, but rather to increase your medical knowledge so that you will take better care of your body. When questions arise, see your physician right away.

I hope readers will enjoy and learn while reading this book, but if not, "Take two aspirin, go to bed and call me in the morning."

1 MEDICATIONS

ASPIRIN

Hippocrates, in ancient Greece, advised his feverish patients to chew on the bark of a willow tree. In the 1800's the beneficial ingredient of the bark was found to be salicylic acid, but the drug in pure form was very irritating to the stomach. The Bayer Company of Germany, in 1899, compounded acetylsalicylic acid which had the benefits of salicylic acid but not as many side effects. ASPIRIN was born!

Has it been successful? One hundred TONS of aspirin are consumed annually! If aspirin were discovered today the FDA (Federal Drug Administration) would require a doctor's prescription before you could buy it because of its strong effects and possible dangers. The three common uses of aspirin are to reduce fever, pain, and arthritis. Scientifically it is an antipyretic (against fever), an analgesic (against pain), and an anti-inflammatory (against swelling) agent. In fact, it has been so effective in these actions that it is used as a standard for comparison of new drugs as they are developed—and few have surpassed aspirin.

A more recently discovered benefit, and dangerous side effect, is aspirin's ability to delay clotting of the blood. This is called an antithrombotic effect, which means that it prevents the blood platelets from sticking to each other and starting the blood clot. This property has been used by doctors in attempts to decrease the numbers of repeated heart attacks, strokes, and blood clots in the legs. The FDA has approved the professional labeling of aspirin "to reduce the risk of death and/or non-fatal myocardial infarction (heart attacks) in patients with a previous infarction or unstable angina pectoris (heart pains)." A single buffered aspirin a day is the recommended dose.

A six-year study to determine the benefits of aspirin in preventing heart attacks, in men who had not yet had one, was completed in 1988 by Dr. Charles Hennekens of Harvard Medical School. The "guinea pigs" were 22,071 U.S. doctors across our country. I was one of the three on Maui. Every other day we would take a "white pill" which was either a buffered aspirin or a placebo (sugar pill). No one knew what they were taking until the six-year study was completed.

In the study there were 99 non-fatal heart attacks among the 11,000 physicians taking the aspirin every other day. However, there were almost TWICE as many (171) non-fatal heart attacks among the other 11,000 who were taking the "sugar pills." Fatal heart attacks were three times as frequent among those taking only the placebo (sugar pill). Fortunately, I learned that I was taking the aspirin.

These results have led to the recommendation that "healthy" men, 40 years or older, should consider taking an aspirin every other day AFTER CONSULTING WITH THEIR PHYSICIAN.

However, the antithrombotic effect is also the cause of aspirin's major danger—bleeding from the stomach. Not only can aspirin, which is an acid, cause ulcers and gastritis (severe irritation of the stomach), but if the ulcer starts to bleed, the aspirin also interferes with the body's attempt to form a clot and stop the bleeding. Because of delayed clotting, patients should not take aspirin the week before elective surgery and pregnant women should avoid aspirin during their final weeks of pregnancy. Patients who are taking Coumadin (a blood thinner) MUST avoid aspirin as the combination of the two drugs can result in dangerous bleeding.

Recently, the Surgeon General has advised that children and teenagers not be given aspirin during attacks of influenza or chickenpox because of a possible association with a disease known as Reye's Syndrome. This disease is rare, difficult to diagnose and possibly fatal. Fortunately, substitutes such as Tylenol, or other brands of acetaminophen, are excellent for children with fever, and will avoid this risk of contracting Reye's Syndrome.

Aspirin is an important drug and must be used with intelligence by both the patient and the doctor. Perhaps now you will have a better understanding the next time you hear, "Take two aspirin, go to bed and call me in the morning."

ANTIBIOTICS

The miracles of modern medicine are due in a large degree to the miracles of modern antibiotics. Heart surgery, hip surgery, the healing of pneumonias—all are possible because of modern antibiotics, and they were discovered by accident!

The medicinal value of mold has been known since the time of the Egyptians. Moldy bread was applied to skin eruptions 5,000 years ago! The ancient Chinese treated boils and infected wounds with mold and soy flour poultices. The American Indians and the Middle Age War Lords also used molds for treating war wounds. Then the value of mold was forgotten for several hundred years, and it was left to a Scottish bacteriologist, Alexander Fleming, to rediscover its value—by accident!

In 1928, Dr. Fleming was studying the growth patterns of staphylococcus, the bacteria that causes pimples, boils and a very serious blood infection. His assistant was supposed to cover each growth-dish immediately after preparation, but one was left open for several minutes and the spores (seeds) of the mold Penicillum notatum, carried by the wind, landed in the dish and began to grow. The staphylococcus bacteria grew abundantly in each dish except the one with the Penicillum mold growing in it. Dr. Fleming noted that around each colony of mold there was a clear area in the broth where the staph could not grow. He believed that the fungus had released a deadly substance into the broth which prevented the staph from multiplying. Being a scientist, Dr. Fleming advanced his discovery further and showed that Penicillum was lethal against not only staphylococcus but also pneumococcus, gonococcus, streptococcus, and a number of other bacteria. But then Dr. Fleming went on to other investigations and Penicillum was forgotten for ten years.

In 1941, Dr. Florey, a British scientist, was able to extract a small amount of penicillin from the mold and showed that it was extremely beneficial in treating infections in man. As World War II was beginning and there was a critical need for this new miracle drug, American scientists became involved in its production. A new strain of Penicillum, from rotten cantaloupes, produced one-hundred times as much penicillin as did Dr. Fleming's strain. Even more important, the Americans found that it would grow more quickly in corn-steep liquor than in previous nutrients. The combined efforts of British and American scientists in developing penicillin saved hundreds of thousands of lives during WW II and millions of lives since then. In 1945, Drs. Fleming and Florey received the Nobel Prize for their discoveries.

After the beneficial effects of the Penicillum mold were realized, every "square mile of the world" was checked for additional medicinal molds. From these investigations came the antibiotics Streptomycin (from the fungus Streptomyces griseus) and Chloramphenicol (from Streptomyces venezuelae).

Next, the scientists in the laboratories began making synthetic penicillins and penicillin-like antibiotics. The cephalosporin antibiotics fall into this category and physicians must now learn about the "third generation" cephalosporins.

What a difference antibiotics have made! Patients no longer lose their legs, arms or lives from "blood poisoning." The injured are able to be saved because the infections can be controlled. Modern surgery is performing miracles because infections can be prevented. Now it is a rare patient who dies from pneumonia. And all because of an accident—and a very inquiring mind!

CALCIUM— ESSENTIAL TO OUR BODIES

Calcium, one of the essential minerals in our body, has become a popular subject. Do we have too much or too little, and what are the consequences? In grade school we learned that calcium "is the cement of the bones" and that if we did not drink milk, our leg bones were going to bow (as in rickets). The importance of calcium goes far beyond the bones as it is involved in most of the physiology (workings) of your body.

Calcium's "claim to fame" is that it changes the electrical properties of the wall of the cells of our body. There are billions of these microscopic cells, and calcium affects each one's permeability (what goes in and out of the cell). Too little calcium (hypocalcemia) increases the cell wall's permeability and increases the activity of the cell, while an excess of calcium (hypercalcemia) decreases its activity. This important delicate balance is maintained by a number of interacting factors: the calcium and vitamin D that we ingest; the functioning of tiny parathyroid glands in our neck; the calcium deposited in our bones; and finally, the action of healthy kidneys.

A low level of calcium in the blood can cause many distressing symptoms. Remember that a LOW calcium level causes an INCREASED activity of the cell. Therefore, with the nervous system (brain and nerves), there is confusion, anxiety, emotional lability and tingling in the hands and feet. Muscles may develop aches and spasms, while, in the intestinal tract, there may be vomiting and diarrhea.

The major cause of hypocalcemia (low calcium) is dietary. This includes people allergic to dairy products, alcoholics with inadequate diets, and individuals with chronic starvation. Other causes include prolonged diarrhea, surgery where the parathyroid glands have been removed, resistance to vitamin D, and kidney failure.

An excess of calcium in the blood also produces undesirable

effects. Remember again that a HIGH calcium level causes a DECREASED activity in the body's cells. Apathy, depression, coma, muscle weakness, heart failure, bone cysts, bone pain and constipation are some of the symptoms. The causes of a high serum calcium include: excessive intake of calcium and vitamin D, tumors of the parathyroid glands, prolonged immobilization, and cancer which has spread to the bones.

The delicate calcium balance in our bodies is another example of the marvelous human machine. It is important not to abuse it with starvation diets or excessive vitamins.

DIGITALIS

My grandfather's medical bag is proudly displayed in a glass case on my desk. The bag is probably 90 years old (Dr. Seagley died in 1910), and it is showing its years. Last week, when I opened the glass case, the medical odors penetrated my office and stirred childhood memories of playing with the bag. The labels are peeling off the old glass vials, but some are still legible. The vial with the purple crystals is labeled "Potassium iodide." Others are: Dover's powder, Fowler's solution, Tincture of Belladona, Boric acid, Sodium salicylate and Tincture of digitalis. Most of grandfather's medicines have been replaced by modern drugs, but digitalis remains one of today's most important therapies.

Digitalis belongs to a group of drugs known as cardiac glycosides, which are extremely important in the treatment of heart failure. Why does a heart fail? If your hands had to squeeze a bag of blood 80 times a minute, 4,800 times an hour, 115,200 times a day, 42,048,000 times a year for 70 or 80 years, your hands would also tire and fail. Digitalis and the other cardiac glycosides reverse heart failure by increasing the force of "myocardial contraction;" that is, it makes the heart muscle squeeze strongly again.

Digitalis is derived from the dried leaf of the foxglove plant—Digitalis purpurea. It was mentioned in the writings of Welsh physicians in 1250. Other cardiac glycosides were known to the ancient Egyptians, Romans and Chinese. For centuries one of man's greatest illnesses was "dropsy," an accumulation of fluid in the lungs, abdomen and legs. The cause was not known, but it was known that a small amount of the leaf of the foxglove plant would cause the fluid "to flow from the body." Unfortunately, because some physicians in the Middle Ages prescribed an excessive amount of the drug, their patients died. As a result, the drug fell from use, except among peasants.

In 1785, it was the work and writings of Dr. William Withering (no relation) that revived the use of digitalis, still known as foxglove. He had founded a clinic for the poor where he treated 3,000 patients a year. Many of these had "dropsy" and he tested the amount of foxglove necessary to relieve their condition. As he increased the dosages, he discovered the symptoms of toxicity, or over-dosage. His writings are still valid today: "The foxglove when given in very large doses occasions sickness, vomiting, confused vision, objects appear green or yellow, slow pulse, cold sweats, convulsions, syncope and death."

Today it is known that the main pharmacodynamic property (why it works) of digitalis is its ability to increase the force of myocardial (heart muscle) contraction. From this comes a decrease in heart size, an increase in cardiac output, decreased venous pressure, increased kidney output and a relief of edema (the modern term for "dropsy"). Grandfather would be impressed with today's cardiac (heart) medications of digoxin, calcium blockers and beta-blockers. But he would still issue the warning: "If you fail to take your medication faithfully, the dropsy will get you."

SILVADENE AND DR. FOX

Last Saturday my wife and I had dinner with Dr. and Mrs. Charles Fox who were visiting from New York. Dr. Fox is a world renowned expert on the treatment of burns, and Carole and I felt honored to have spent the evening with him. Very few modern-day physicians ever make original contributions to the advancement of medicine. We rely upon the brilliant researchers who have gone before us. Dr. Fox is one of those rare men, and his discovery of a true "miracle drug" for the treatment of burns has saved thousands of lives world-wide.

Twenty years ago burns were treated with sulfa drugs or solutions of silver nitrate. All of these medications had serious drawbacks. Dr. Fox, in his research laboratory at Columbia University, New York, experimented by mixing many combinations of silver nitrate with different sulfa drugs.

Using anesthetized burned mice, he treated their burns with his different mixtures until he found one that worked best. After months of experimenting, a miracle drug, code name CF-100, was refined. Next the drug was used in tests on human patients, and the early results were published in the surgical journal, *Archives of Surgery*, (Feb., 1968). It was in this publication that I first read about Dr. Fox's outstanding results.

At about this time I was called to see an eight-month-old child who had suffered severe coffee burns on his face and back. The bacteria pseudomonas was growing extensively on the burns of the skin and was resistant to the drugs being used. I called Dr. Fox in New York, and he sent a case of CF-100 by air freight. It arrived on Maui the next morning. The child's grandmother, who had been staying with him in the hospital, was overjoyed when, within six hours of using this new medicine, her grandson was freed of pain and able to sleep. Today he is an adult and has no scars!

Dr. Fox asked if the physicians at Maui Memorial Hospital would join in a national study to evaluate CF-100. When the medical staff agreed, several cases of CF-100 were shipped to us.

The next month I was called to see the worst burn patient ever treated at our hospital. A Pioneer Mill worker, whose clothing had caught on fire, sustained burns to 50% of his body, including his face, arms, hands, abdomen, back and legs. In addition to large amounts of intravenous fluids, he required daily trips to the operating room to change his burn dressings. Many cases of CF-100 were used during these treatments. The patient progressed steadily and, after skin grafting and physical therapy, was able to walk upright and happy when he left the hospital. Eventually he returned to normal health and resumed his work.

Our hospital's tabulations on these CF-100 cases and several others, added to the hundreds of cases across the United States, led the Federal Drug Administration to approve the drug which is now marketed under the name "Silvadene." It is now the leading burn medication world-wide.

Considering the thousands of lives that have been saved by this drug, I believe that the lives of the laboratory mice, while not given voluntarily, were not in vain. I asked Dr. Fox if he would like to establish a research laboratory in Kihei where millions of mice migrate every four years. He replied, "There could be no lovelier place to do research."

Dr. Fox, welcome to Maui. There are several Mauians who owe you their lives. Thank you.

2 HEALTH HABITS

CHOLESTEROL AND ITS DANGERS

Do you live to eat, or eat to live? In our modern society of McDonald's hamburgers, TV dinners and an occasional "night out," eating has become convenient, tasty and glorious—but it could also be dangerous to your health!

There are over 500,000 deaths each YEAR from heart attacks in the United States! More than another 500,000 persons who have had a heart attack survive but require surgery or medication for the rest of their lives. Evidence is now available which shows that arteriosclerosis of the coronary (heart) arteries—the cause of heart attacks—is not a natural process of life. In fact, it is something which we do to ourselves, so we CAN PREVENT IT FROM OCCURRING!

There are several risk factors for heart attacks we cannot modify and therefore must live with. For example, heart attacks are more common in men, but the rate in women climbs after menopause. Fortunately, women can obtain protection by taking estrogens. In addition, with increasing age the incidence of heart attacks increases, but this risk can be reduced by taking better care of our bodies through the years. At times, an elevated cholesterol can be hereditary, so a family history of heart attacks is extremely important in determining your risk. Because my mother, her father and her brother died of heart attacks, I have become acutely aware of watching my diet, getting exercise and reducing my cholesterol level.

You cannot change your sex, the fact that you are growing older, or your family background, so what *can* you change in order to decrease your risk of having a heart attack? Hypertension, smoking, lack of exercise, diabetes, obesity and an elevated blood cholesterol are all factors which will increase your risk. These you *can* do something about!

At this point, a definition of terms will clarify any confusion you may have about cholesterol. Actually, cholesterol is the sum of three lipoproteins (fat-carrying proteins) in the blood. One of the lipoproteins is healthful, but the other two are very bad for you. Low-density lipoprotein (LDL) is believed to be the most dangerous. This protein carries the fatty cholesterol through the blood stream and deposits it on the wall of the artery which finally becomes plugged, and causes the heart attack. Very-low-density lipoprotein (VLDL) is used by the liver to produce LDL, so too much of this in your blood is also bad. But there is good news with high-density lipoprotein (HDL). This protein carries the fatty cholesterol AWAY FROM the vessels and acts as a protection from heart attacks. The formula to remember is: total cholesterol= LDL + HDL + VLDL.

This leads to another important number—the total cholesterol/HDL ratio. Since HDL is a protective protein, the more the HDL, or the lower the ratio, the better. If your doctor tells you that your ratio is 3.5, go out and celebrate by ordering a good steak dinner.

All this information is of no value if YOU do not KNOW your cholesterol, LDL and HDL levels. It is now recommended that every male over the age of 20 should have a blood test, and know his "levels," and modify his life style IF necessary. Women who are past menopause, or have a family history of heart disease, should also know these levels.

If your cholesterol is below 200 and your ratio is under four, you exercise regularly, have no family history of heart attacks and do not smoke, read no further. Go out and eat the foods you enjoy. But if you are like the majority of Americans, read on and you may learn some tips which will decrease your risk of having a heart attack. As an example, only a year ago my cholesterol had risen to 261. It is now 165. If I can do it—you can!

DIET AND CHOLESTEROL

If you are a male over 20 years of age, or a woman past menopause, you should know your cholesterol, HDL and LDL levels. If your cholesterol is greater than 200, the LDL greater than 130 or the cholesterol/HDL ratio greater than five, then changes are necessary in your eating habits in order to decrease your risks of having a heart attack.

All dietary experts (I do not consider myself one) agree that the first way to attack a high blood cholesterol level is to change one's diet by decreasing the amount of cholesterol and fat that is ingested.

Fats are divided into saturated, monounsaturated and polyunsaturated according to the molecular bonds indicating the saturation of carbon atoms. Saturated fats, after being absorbed, will raise the cholesterol and LDL levels in the blood. They are found in all red meats (beef, lamb, ham), whole milk dairy products (cheese, butter, ice cream), coconut, palm oils and cocoa butter. Monounsaturated fatty acids are found in nuts and seeds, avocados, olives, olive oil and natural peanut butter. These fatty acids tend to help in lowering the total cholesterol and LDL. The "best" fatty acids are the polyunsaturated ones which are present in liquid vegetable oils and fish. These are definitely protective in lowering total cholesterol and LDL.

Ingested cholesterol is dangerous for many people, and for every 100mg eaten (one egg yolk has 250 mg) the blood cholesterol will be raised five to seven mg.

The American diet has been criticized as having too many calories, too much fat (50% of the calories), not enough fiber, and too much cholesterol. A "Quarter Pounder" with cheese and French fries will give you 729 calories, 40 gms of fat (saturated), 109 mg of cholesterol and little fiber. A "healthy" diet for a 150 pound active man for a WHOLE DAY is 2,250 calories, 50 gms of fat (unsaturated), 250 mg cholesterol and plenty of fiber.

There are numerous diet books available which will help you determine a healthy diet for your size, age and activity level. I highly recommend *The 8-Week Cholesterol Cure* (Harper and Row, 1987) by Robert E. Kowalski. It has been a best seller for many months and the hints and advice given by Mr. Kowalski have worked for me.

When you start on your low cholesterol diet you will want to learn the grams of fat and mgms of cholesterol in each of your foods. For the present, however, it is enough to know these foods are good for you: skim milk, low fat yogurt, chicken and turkey (without skin), beans, peas, egg whites, tuna canned in water, fish, whole grain breads and cereals, baked potatoes, all vegetables, all fruit, and for dessert—angel food cake. Unfortunately, the list of the foods bad for you is longer and includes: whole milk, ice cream, butter, most cheeses, egg yolk, red meats, doughnuts and most baked goods, coconut, chocolate and caramel. As a special warning, avoid coconut as it contains 92% saturated fat, or TWICE as much as beef! Unfortunately, I love coconut cream pie, but it may be many years before I enjoy it again, if ever.

A low fat, low cholesterol diet is only the start of lowering the cholesterol in your blood. Begin today to alter your dietary habits to achieve a longer life.

MEDICATIONS AND THE CONTROL OF CHOLESTEROL

Now you know that eating the bacon and eggs you love for breakfast and enjoying the coconut doughnut for a snack are the wrong ways to reduce your cholesterol below the 200 level. Then what are the correct ways to maintain an acceptable cholesterol level?

Medical science is spending millions of dollars to develop the perfect PILL to lower your cholesterol, protect you from heart attacks and yet allow you to eat all that you want—with no side effects from taking the magic pill. So far they are falling short of the goal. Even the drug companies emphasize that a low cholesterol diet is the first important step in lowering your cholesterol. To remember the foods which are good and bad for you, let your conscience be your guide.

If the diet is not successful, then several medications are available to help. The medications can be broadly classified as those that act in the intestine by holding onto the cholesterol and fats, and those that act on the liver by interfering with the production of cholesterol and increasing its excretion or removal. Both groups have side effects, but those that act on the liver are more dangerous.

One of the body's natural uses of cholesterol is that it is made into bile acids which are excreted by the liver into the intestine, assisting in the absorption of fats. The bile and cholesterol are then reabsorbed by the body to be used again. Two medications bind onto the bile and prevent it and the cholesterol from this natural reabsorption. With these medications the bile is excreted with the feces. If enough bile is removed by this method, the cholesterol level in the blood will start to decline. Unfortunately, these medications (cholestyramine and colestipol) can cause constipation, abdominal cramps, gallstones, gallbladder disease and arthritis. Cholestyramine is also expensive, costing about $80/month.

The other group of medications, those that act in the liver, can be very effective but also very dangerous. Lopid (gemfibrozil) is effective in elevating HDL (the good cholesterol) and decreasing triglycerides, but it can cause an increased number of infections in the gallbladder and pancreas and is associated with an increase in cancer deaths. Mevacor (lovastatin) blocks an enzyme (chemical) in the liver which is necessary for the production of cholesterol.

It drastically lowers the blood cholesterol in the patient taking the medication, but it has also been blamed for muscle cramps, cataracts, and even kidney failure.

There are, however, more natural ways to control your cholesterol. They are described by Robert E. Kowalski in *The 8-Week Cholesterol Cure*. The author had his first heart attack at age 35, requiring a coronary bypass operation, then a second operation on his heart at age 41. He decided that if he were to live to see his children grow up, he had to control his cholesterol and prevent further damage to his coronary arteries. Being a professional medical writer, he had access to all the medical reports he needed. Medications to absorb the fat in the intestine and drugs to block the production of cholesterol in the liver were not acceptable to Mr. Kowalski, so he looked for other scientifically proven methods which would be more palatable to him. A low cholesterol diet was his first step, and he strived for the recommended goal of a diet with only 20% of the calories from fat (unsaturated) and a daily cholesterol of only 250 mg (the equivalent of one egg yolk).

His readings tipped him off to the value of oat bran in absorbing the cholesterol in the intestine and how niacin (a B vitamin you can buy without a prescription) blocks production of cholesterol in the liver. With his diet, oat bran muffins and daily niacin, Mr. Kowalski's cholesterol level dropped from 284 mg/dl to a healthy 169. When he shared his findings with physicians and other high risk individuals, their results were equally as good.

His book started the "oat bran craze," and I am sure that he has prevented hundreds, if not thousands, of heart attacks and deaths.

OAT BRAN vs. CHOLESTEROL

If you have been faithful to your low fat-low cholesterol diet and your doctor tells you that your serum cholesterol is still over 200, then the next step is to consider adding oat bran to your diet.

Anyone who has watched the breakfast cereal ads on TV for the last several years has heard that there are benefits to eating fiber ever day. Certainly, fiber will keep your bowels regular, but it can also help lower your cholesterol! Fifteen years ago, Dr. Dennis Burkitt reported that civilizations which ate high fiber diets also had low blood cholesterol and low rates of heart attacks.

But all fiber types are not equal in lowering cholesterol. Wheat bran has three times as much insoluble fiber as does oat bran, but oat bran has four times as much soluble fiber. It is the soluble fraction that does the work in reducing the cholesterol levels. The exact way that oat bran does this is not fully understood; however, when oat bran is ingested, bile acids from the liver increase and are excreted into the intestine, which removes cholesterol from the body. This action is similar to the actions of the drugs colestipol and cholestyramine, but without their side effects or expense.

Oat bran lowers the total cholesterol and the damaging LDL fraction, but it does not reduce the beneficial HDL fraction. This is not the only good news about oat bran. It supplies six gm of protein per serving plus many vitamins and minerals. It practically guarantees to keep your stools regular and will also help you lose those extra pounds around your waist. The weight loss results not only from the fats being absorbed by the oat bran and excreted in the stool, but after eating oat bran in the morning, you do not feel hungry until into the afternoon. There is no need for snacking.

Now that the value of eating oat bran is understood, how do you eat the 1/2 cup of oat bran to meet the daily requirement? Hot cereal is probably the fastest but not the tastiest way. Adding brown sugar or honey helps the taste. The best way to use the oat bran is to bake muffins and add apple slices, pineapple or banana—but never coconut. Three muffins a day will fulfill what you need. What a tasty way to reduce your cholesterol! I usually have two muffins for breakfast and the third as a snack in the late morning. How much healthier than a donut!

The 8-Week Cholesterol Cure provides oat bran recipes for delicious muffins, dinner rolls, breads, and brownies. Included also are low cholesterol recipes for fixing turkey, turkeyburgers, pizzas, meatballs and many other foods. As Mr. Kowalski avows, "You don't have to give up eating to live."

NIACIN vs. CHOLESTEROL

If you are a male over 20, or a woman past menopause, then you should know your serum cholesterol level. If it is under 200 mg/dl and you exercise regularly, do not smoke and no one in your family has had a heart attack—read no further. You will probably live to a "ripe old age"—laughing at those of us who have to fight the "cholesterol battle."

The previous articles have described the cholesterol components in your blood and their dangerous levels. We learned about foods high in saturated fats and cholesterol which should be avoided. The value of oat bran and the ways to incorporate it in our diets were also noted. Now let's discuss the benefits of niacin.

Seventy years ago niacin, a B vitamin, was known to cure the rare disease, pellagra. It was not until 1955 that niacin was also found to reduce cholesterol. Since that time there have been numerous medical reports confirming the benefit of this "over-the-counter" vitamin. A report in the *Journal of the American Medical Association* (June 19, 1987) compared 162 men with previous coronary bypass surgery. All of the men had a coronary angiogram (an X-ray of the arteries of the heart) and were placed on a low fat diet. Then half were also given the drug colestipol (which binds the bile-acids in the bowel) and large doses of niacin, while the other half of the men were given only a placebo (sugar pill). After two years, all the men received a second angiogram and had their cholesterol levels tested. The results were amazing! In the group taking the niacin and colestipol, there was a 26% reduction in total cholesterol, a 43% reduction in LDL (the bad cholesterol) and a 37% increase in HDL (the good cholesterol). The best news, however, was that there was only 1/4 the number of recurrent heart attacks (one) in the group taking the niacin and colestipol as compared to the group taking the sugar pill. In addition, x-rays showed that the plugging of the heart arteries had actually DECREASED in 16% of the group which used niacin. This study showed for the first time that arteriosclerosis is REVERSIBLE!

Niacin appears to act in the liver by blocking the production of VLDL (very-low density lipoprotein) and decreasing the level of LDL (the bad cholesterol). Equally important is that niacin increases the HDL (high density lipoprotein), the good cholesterol. So it is a "win-win" situation.

Robert Kowalski's *The 8-Week Cholesterol Cure* describes in detail the benefits and complications of niacin therapy. His recommendation is to add 1,500 mg daily to your diet—BUT ONLY AFTER YOU HAVE TALKED TO YOUR DOCTOR.

The prescription drugs Lopid and Mevacor, which also act on the liver, can have serious side effects, BUT SO CAN NIACIN. The most common complaint of someone taking niacin is a warm sensation or a "flush." This is usually not noticed when a person takes "time-released" niacin. Abnormalities of liver tests, activation of ulcers and gout are rare, but significant, and you should ask your family physician before taking any niacin.

Now you have all the information you need to lower your cholesterol: 1) KNOW your cholesterol; 2) If your cholesterol is over 200, the first step is to begin a low fat, low cholesterol diet and stick to it for several months; 3) If the cholesterol remains over 200, add 1/2 cup of oat bran daily to your diet to help lower your level; 4) After a couple months, if your level is still not below 200, then see your doctor about taking 1,500 mg of niacin daily (or another medication).

These four steps have worked for me, and I know that they can work for you. Good luck, good eating, GOOD HEALTH!

THE DANGERS OF SMOKING

As I drove to Kihei I laughed when I read the bumper sticker on the car in front of me: "CANCER CURES SMOKING." This is certainly true if the cancer wins and the patient finally dies. In contrast, if surgery wins and the patient is cured, the addiction to nicotine may be so strong that, in spite of having a second chance at life, the patient begins smoking again! Unbelievable? Unfortunately not.

Last week Gerald came into my office for his monthly checkup. A year ago I had operated and removed part of his left lung in the hope of curing an early carcinoma. The cancer was the result of 30 years of smoking cigarettes. As I walked into the exam room Gerald greeted me with, "Yes." My reply was, "Yes—what?" Gerald said, "Yes, I am smoking again and I know that it is wrong, but I just can't help it." As his doctor I became upset because I knew that Gerald would be "inhaling" his death warrant. The more I thought about his problem, the more I realized Gerald was not alone. Of the many patients I have operated on for lung cancer, all but two started smoking again. Ironically, they all knew smoking had caused their cancers and they were aware of the risks they were taking.

It is next to impossible for an older adult to give up smoking. So, for the younger adults who want to stop smoking, and to the parents who want to help their children avoid smoking, I want to emphasize the risks that one takes when deciding to smoke cigarettes.

The American Cancer Society estimates that 139,000 Americans died from lung cancer in 1988. Eighty-five percent (85%) of these deaths are the direct result of smoking cigarettes. The U.S. Surgeon General, Dr. C. Everett Koop, reports that a person who smokes more than one pack a day has three times the chance of a non-smoker of dying from cancer (lung or other types). Cigarette smoking is not only implicated in causing lung cancer, but it also causes cancers of the mouth, larynx (voice box), esophagus, kidney and urinary bladder.

While smoking causes 30% of all cancers, it is also a major cause of heart disease, emphysema, chronic bronchitis and ulcers. It is estimated that smoking is directly related to 320,000 deaths each year. Dr. Koop declares that cigarette smoking is "the chief, single, avoidable cause of death in our society, and the most important health issue of our time."

So why, with all this frightening evidence, do people such as

Gerald (who has faced death) go back to smoking? Even more serious, why do physicians, who deal with cancer deaths daily, continue to smoke? The answer is not complex: nicotine addiction is one of the strongest addictions man has discovered. It ranks with cocaine addiction. In fact, breaking the smoking habit takes months, and sometimes years, and yet the overall success rate is only 10% to 50%!

With the risks from smoking so high and the cures so low, the best way to deal with smoking is never to start. I applaud the grade school teachers who stress to our young children the health risks of smoking. High school teachers must follow through and not allow smoking on campus. Cigarette advertising must be stopped, parents must become involved, programs to quit smoking must be expanded, and smoking should be banned in all public areas.

A week before Christmas I examined a patient who was in his final painful months from lung cancer. He had had x-ray treatment and chemotherapy because his cancer was advanced at the time of its discovery. I will never be able to forget his first office visit. After I showed him the large cancer on the x-ray, he commented, "Well, they got me, doc." "Who got you?" I replied. "The coffin nails—the cigarettes," he answered.

He was right. "CANCER CURES SMOKING." Although true, why don't YOU cure your smoking habits before it is too late?

SMOKING: WAYS TO QUIT

Pointing to the x-ray, I said, "I'm sorry to tell you, but you have lung cancer and will need an operation to remove part of your lung. This is all that we can do for you at this time. You have a 20% chance of being alive in five years." Harsh words but true.

If you are a smoker I could have been talking to you. If you smoke and have children, another doctor could be telling this to them in forty years. Would you like to change this grim prediction?

Then read on and I will try to help you abandon the cigarette habit.

There are only two reasons why a person begins to smoke. The first is that one or both parents smoke and the child learns "this is the way to live and my father knows more than the doctor." The second reason is that peer pressure motivates adolescents to begin smoking. Their friends smoke because it is "the thing to do."

Studies in high schools have shown that students who do well in their studies and in athletics are those who do not "need to smoke." Others, searching for some type of recognition, "join the gang" and begin a habit that will affect them the rest of their lives.

Smoking, as an unhealthy habit, should be addressed more vigorously in the grade schools and high schools. If children can avoid the smoking habit during these years, they will probably be able to avoid it altogether.

Once the smoker is "hooked," there are several reasons for continuing to smoke: relaxation, release of tensions, craving a cigarette or pure chemical addiction.

For true cigarette addicts it is necessary to go through two withdrawals to break the habit. The first stage is physical withdrawal, which may take five to seven days. This may include severe headaches, irritability, muscle aches, cramps, anxiety, insomnia and an intense craving for tobacco. Some individuals can "cold turkey" the habit and have no symptoms whatsoever. The second stage of withdrawal is psychological and can last weeks or years. During this time the individual can think of hundreds of reasons not to give up smoking: fear of gaining weight, expecting to fail, a fear of being unable to cope with stressful situations, etc....

For those of you who wish to stop smoking, here are some helpful suggestions:

1. Actively help others to stop smoking.
2. Seek out your friends who were former smokers and get their help.
3. Throw away all cigarettes, cigarette holders, and other paraphernalia that remind you of smoking.

4. Attend a quit-smoking clinic and share your problems with others.

5. Make a cash bet with a close friend so that you will have a monetary goal in kicking your habit.

6. Take up a sport or other physical activity, such as running, dancing, aerobics or long-distance walking to help you develop a better lung capacity.

7. Ask your doctor to give you a prescription for Nicorettes, a nicotine substitute, to help you through the early stages of withdrawal.

Information on quit-smoking clinics can be obtained by calling the American Lung Association. Make every effort to stop smoking in order to improve your own health. Even more important, however, is to set a good example for your children. Help them avoid this deadly danger to their health.

COFFEE AND CAFFEINE

Eight hundred years ago, Ethiopian goatherders noticed that their flocks stayed awake at night after eating the leaves and berries of a small tree. The goatherders made a drink from the berries and coffee was discovered. The world has been on a caffeine high ever since.

There are many controversies about the benefits and side effects of caffeine and coffee, and I thought you might be interested in some facts on this subject. The best scientific article I could find is entitled "The Health Consequences of Caffeine" by Peter Curatolo M.D. and David Robertson M.D., published in *Annals of Internal Medicine* (May 1985). The authors report not only on their own findings, but also combine them with the findings from 281 other scientific articles.

Caffeine is the most frequently studied chemical in coffee, but there are hundreds of others. One of these is chlorogenic acid, which may have detrimental effects on our bodies. There are many conflicting reports on caffeine's effects because it acts very differently in chronic users (heavy coffee drinkers) and occasional users.

Caffeine's effects on the heart can be critical. In non-coffee drinkers caffeine will increase the blood pressure and the heart rate. Interestingly, this is not the reaction with the chronic coffee drinker. Two studies showed a twofold increase of heart attacks in people who drink more than six cups of coffee daily. However, many recent investigations have failed to support this finding. Who is correct? It IS known that caffeine increases the incidence of premature ventricular contractions (extra heart beats) and cardiac arrhythmias (irregular heart beats) in susceptible persons.

For the last forty years caffeine has been known to increase the acid and the pepsin in the stomach. Recently it was shown that coffee and decaffeinated coffee produced more acid than caffeine alone. The obvious conclusion is that individuals with ulcers should drink neither regular nor decaffeinated coffee.

As it did with the goats in Ethiopia, coffee interferes with human sleep. Caffeine delays sleep, decreases total sleep time and diminishes the "quality" of sleep. Its effect on mood is variable. Non-drinkers of coffee report anxiety and nervousness while chronic coffee drinkers report "pleasant stimulation" and alertness—the morning "pick-me-up" reported by coffee users. Although caffeine can decrease the muscular response time to stimuli, it has no significant reversal of the depressant effect of alcohol. What this means is that coffee will NOT improve your driving if you have had too much to drink.

During the last five years, doctors have advised women with fibrocystic disease of the breasts to avoid all caffeine. Presently the studies which recommended this advice are under scrutiny and are believed to be in error. As a surgeon, I personally have not been impressed with any improvement in the symptoms from fibrocystic disease as a result of avoiding caffeine.

Can coffee cause cancer? Many studies have shown that there is no relationship between drinking coffee and cancer of the urinary bladder or kidney, but cancer of the pancreas may be another matter. In 1981, Dr. MacMahon reported in the *New England Journal of Medicine* that there was a threefold increase of cancer of the pancreas in individuals who drank five cups of coffee a day. This caused considerable alarm and was reported on national TV news. The study was shown to have some flaws, but other studies also suggested a cause and effect. More investigation is being conducted concerning this very serious medical problem.

As a young man I was able to consume many cups of coffee daily, but as I grew older, coffee interfered with my sleep—just like those Ethiopian goats. Today my wife is happy that I switched to decaffeinated coffee. She says that I became more "pleasant" but, like wine, maybe I mellowed with age.

FISH

Fish—the food for longevity? A scientific report in *The New England Journal of Medicine* (May 9, 1985) would lead us to believe this. For years it had been known that the Eskimos and the Japanese have very low rates of heart attacks and consume large amounts of fish. Are these two circumstances related? The report deals with 872 Dutch men, ages 40 to 59, who were followed for 20 years to determine their dietary habits and their rate of heart attacks. The results were startling!

The average fish consumption per man was 20 grams per day; however, 20% of the men ate no fish at all. Of the fish eaten, 2/3 were lean fish (cod) while 1/3 was fatty fish (herring and mackerel). Seventy-eight men died of heart attacks during the twenty year period. Their life styles were closely studied as to age, fish consumption, dietary cholesterol, blood pressure, serum cholesterol, cigarette smoking, obesity, physical activity, caloric intake, and occupation. Only age, dietary cholesterol and fish consumption showed any relation to heart attacks. In fact, the older one becomes, or the more animal fat (cholesterol) that is eaten, the greater the risk of having a heart attack. But the more one eats fish, the lower the risk. For example, the fatal heart attack rate was cut 50% by eating only 30 grams of fish per day, or about two fish dishes per week.

How does this "protection" occur? In this study there was no reduction in the serum cholesterol among the men who ate the 30 grams of fish per day. However, the Eskimos (who eat 400 grams of fish per day) have very low levels of cholesterol and triglycerides. High fish oil diets are known to reduce high triglyceride levels which are especially dangerous for women in developing heart attacks.

The authors of the article believe that the "protection" comes from "omega 3" polyunsaturated fatty acid found in fish. This substance reduces platelet aggregation (blood clotting) and increases bleeding time. A similar reaction is found by taking an aspirin every day.

With all the delicious fish available to us from Hawaiian waters, we should have a low incidence of heart attacks, but that is not the case. I asked a Hawaiian patient why, and she replied, "Too much poi and pig, and not enough fish—it costs too much."

HINTS FOR TOURISTS

As the snow falls and the temperatures dip to minus ten degrees on the Mainland, many visitors arrive on Maui to share in our wonderful weather, waves and hospitality. We are happy to see you arrive, and offer these health hints about the sun and the sea so that you can avoid some injuries that could spoil your vacation.

The most common injury a visitor may suffer is from the sun. Granted, it is a sign of failure to leave Hawaii without a good tan, but how you go about getting it is very important. Even in the winter months the sun's reflection off the waves can cause severe second degree burns. It is recommended that you buy and USE a sun screen lotion with a PABA rating of 10-15. Apply it often during the first several days to all exposed parts. Also, limit your exposure to the sun the first few days and you will be able to leave Hawaii with a good tan rather than with bandages!

The greatest danger to visitors year after year has been those beautiful waves crashing on our beaches. Even our local residents have sustained neck injuries with resulting paralysis of arms and legs when attempting to body surf in the large waves. When they are "pounded" into the sand, they sustain an irreversible injury. Please have great respect for the shoreline and the waves even when not body surfing. A wave can knock you down, fracturing a leg or rupturing the spleen.

We have several spiny creatures in our ocean which we call sea urchins. The sea urchin with long black thin spines is quite dangerous. The spines inject a painful toxin into the skin when they break off and may require surgical removal in the physician's office. Sea urchins with short fuzzy spines or long thick red spines are safe to handle, but why not leave them for others to enjoy viewing?

Occasionally in the winter months, following Kona storms and winds, the small Portuguese man-of-war jellyfish are blown onto Maui's beaches. They look like translucent purple bubbles with long tentacles hanging from them. The Portuguese man-of-war can inflict very painful burning injuries to the arms, legs and chest. A "drug store" treatment for these stings is to apply meat tenderizer or rubbing alcohol in an effort to neutralize the toxins. A cold beer poured over the injury is a good "beach" cure. Frequently, antihistamines and pain medications are necessary.

The beautiful coral heads off Maui's beaches are lovely to look at and best to leave in place. Even minor coral cuts can be troublesome to heal when small particles of coral are left in the skin. If you get a coral cut, scrub it vigorously with soap and water and apply an antibiotic ointment. Even then an infection may occur which will require stronger, oral antibiotics.

The physicians of Maui want you to have a marvelous vacation, enjoy our island, and heed our warnings. Hopefully you can avoid seeing us, but isn't it comforting to know we're here?

DIETING vs. OBESITY SURGERY

The fork or the knife—which will it be? If you are overweight and wish to "lose some of yourself," you must answer that question. It is no longer a question that obesity is dangerous to your health. In fact, it is now well-known that being overweight increases the risks of heart attacks, strokes and cancer. With these forecasts of doom, the decision to lose weight should be easy, but the loss itself is very difficult.

There are two roads for weight loss that might be followed. The first is dieting, also known as "keeping the fork on the table rather than in your mouth." The second is willingly subjecting yourself to a surgeon's knife in a major operation. I will present some up-to-date information on these two methods of weight reduction.

Dieting, or "keeping the fork out of your mouth," is certainly the least expensive and most natural method of losing weight. Many dietary and weight-reduction programs are available and most of them are very well-planned and safe.

Many individuals want a faster solution to their obesity, however, and have followed "near starvation" diets. Although these diets produce results more rapidly, they carry a risk to the individual. Several years ago there was a popular "total protein diet" which resulted in a number of deaths from heart failure. This is one reason for the present warnings from the FDA concerning recent dietary fads. A sensible diet should include the necessary proteins, vitamins and at least 1,000 calories per day.

A common problem of dieters is that they usually develop a habit of "snacking" between meals and, although they may faithfully follow their diets, the "snacks" defeat them.

The other road to weight reduction is surgery. A weight reduction operation is recommended only for those individuals who are at least 100 pounds over their ideal weight, have health problems occurring because of their weight, and have conscientiously tried for at least six months and have failed to lose weight. Because emotional problems frequently need to be overcome before progressing on a surgical course, an evaluation by a psychiatrist is also recommended.

Fifteen years ago the operation of choice was the "intestinal bypass." The small intestine was transected (cut across) several inches past the stomach, and was then anastomosed (reattached) almost at the end of the intestinal tract. Because no intestine was removed in the bypass surgery, it could be hooked up again as nature had originally intended when results were unsuccessful.

With the "intestinal bypass" patients could eat all the food they wanted and it would quickly pass through the few inches of remaining intestine into the large bowel and then into the toilet.

For the patient there was not only the inconvenience of having 6 to 12 or more bowel movements a day, but there was also a significant danger. Frequently the patients developed vitamin deficiencies and liver problems which, in several cases, led to their deaths.

The "intestinal bypass" operation has now been replaced by the "gastric bypass," an operation on the stomach which changes its capacity to hold food. Several types of stomach operations have been utilized during the past ten years. All of these tend to decrease the size of the stomach, from a pouch that can usually hold two quarts of food, down to a smaller pouch that can hold only "two jiggers." When the small stomach is filled with a couple bites of food, the patient has a sensation of being "full" and is no longer hungry.

Psychologically, it may be difficult for these individuals to retrain themselves in their new eating habits and they may require professional counseling. They will find themselves sitting down at the Thanksgiving table to enjoy a large plateful of turkey, dressing, yams and vegetables, but after only two mouthfuls of turkey they will be unable to eat more.

Obesity is not healthy at any age, and a cute, chubby child may grow into an unhappy, overweight adult. A properly supervised diet is the healthiest and least expensive method of regaining one's ideal weight. For the obese individual the choice must remain—the fork or the knife. Which will it be?

3 Cancer

MELANOMA

Dan died two days before his 41st birthday. He had been in the prime years of his life when he discovered a large black mole at his belt line. He let it grow before he had it removed, but by then it was too late. Two years passed before it recurred with a vengeance, and his last year was a day-by-day survival. Before he died, Dan asked me to write about melanoma so that others might be spared his fate.

Malignant melanoma, which appears as a black mole, is the most deadly form of skin cancer. Fortunately 95% of skin cancers are basal cell cancers (usually appearing pearly white) and are easily curable by simple excision. Deaths from basal cell skin cancers are VERY rare, whereas malignant melanoma caused 5,800 deaths in the U.S. during 1988 and the numbers continue to increase every year.

Malignant melanoma can develop from a black mole that has been present for many years or can begin as a cancerous mole. It can occur anywhere on the body, but men's backs and women's legs are the most common areas. We believe the sun can cause them to grow as they are more common in Australia, Hawaii and the "Sun Belt" areas of the Mainland.

When I learned about melanoma in medical school it was considered an almost hopeless form of cancer, and few patients survived more than five years. Most people at that time were unaware of the danger and waited to see their doctor until the mole had grown for many months. By then the melanoma had spread throughout the body.

Now, with better public and medical education, physicians are seeing people with melanomas at an earlier stage and are curing 50-60% of them. BUT THEY CAN DO BETTER. Investigative reports by Dr. Breslow demonstrate that if the melanoma is less than 0.75mm thick (that's 1/2 the thickness of a penny) when it is removed, the cure rate is 100%; however, if a patient waits until the melanoma grows thicker and deeper to more than three mm (the thickness of two quarters), the cure rate falls to 22%.

The life saving facts to remember are: If a mole has changed in size or shape, has developed an irritation, or has begun bleeding—have it removed. If a mole is located in an area which is continually irritated by a belt or clothing—have it removed. If a mole has an irregular border or is colored with shades of black, brown, or blue—have it removed.

Wouldn't you rather have a small scar (I have three) from the removal of a benign mole, rather than risk the surgery, danger and possible death associated with this cancer?

Dan, I hope that the memory of your tragic illness will shock others into having their moles checked. Then perhaps someone will be spared an early and unnecessary death.

COLON CANCER

Cancer of the colon (the large intestine) is never a pleasant subject, but we MUST talk about it again and again if we are ever going to raise people's consciousness and save them from developing this dreaded disease.

Two or three patients a month are operated on at Maui Memorial Hospital for colon cancer. This number of cases only reemphasizes that cancer of the colon, whether we want to talk about it or not, is still one of the most common cancers in the United States, with over 105,000 new cases discovered each year. Half of these patients will die from their cancer because it was discovered too late! We can do much better in saving lives from this frequent cancer if we (physicians and patients) will only discover it earlier.

Colon cancer is a disease of the middle and later years of life, and 95% of the cases occur after the age of fifty. Its causes are thought to be from the foods we eat—meat and fats, and from the foods we do not eat—fiber.

Researchers believe that it takes several years for the cancer to grow from its origin in a polyp (a small benign growth) of the colon until it breaks through the wall of the bowel and spreads to the lymph nodes, liver or lungs. It is during these FEW years that a physician MUST find the cancer and remove it if the patient is to be cured.

Unfortunately, colon cancer is rarely accompanied by early symptoms. The American Cancer Society has publicized the symptoms of "a change in bowel habits," "abdominal pain" and "rectal bleeding" as warnings for colon cancer. Only rectal bleeding may be an early sign, but it can also be a late finding.

So what are people to do if they want to be protected against dying from colon cancer? In an attempt to detect the cancer early, the American Cancer Society recommends that every person over the age of fifty have an annual rectal exam, including a guaiac stool test, with a sigmoidoscopic exam every two years. The guaiac test is inexpensive, painless, and can be done by the patient at home. Although not infallible, it offers the best chance of detecting an early cancer. A positive test does not necessarily mean a cancer is present, but it does mean that additional tests, including a barium enema, are needed. The sigmoidoscopic exam is helpful in detecting cancers in the last twelve to fifteen inches of the bowel. Many doctors now have the newer flexible fiberoptic sigmoidoscope which is less painful than the metal scope and can be advanced farther up the colon in search of early cancers.

Thoughts of colon cancer, guaiac tests and rectal exams may

be unpleasant, but 20-30 people on Maui this year will be diagnosed to have this dreaded cancer. How wonderful it would be if they were all found early enough to be cured!

If you are over 50 and have not had a guaiac test and the other exams this year, take active steps to protect yourself. See your doctor or call the American Cancer Society. Your life may depend on it!

CAROLE'S BREAST CANCER

Ever since my husband began writing the *"Two Aspirin"* column, I have acted as his "at-home-editor," dotting i's, crossing t's and checking verb tenses. But this time I asked to write the article myself. The subject is about something very important to me—BREAST CANCER. I am not a physician and I am only expressing my personal opinions. I am making no attempt to prescribe treatment or diagnosis. All the statistics I use are found in literature supplied by the American Cancer Society.

Recently I was doing breast self-examination (BSE) and I found a small lump that had not been there before. It was that simple and final. John examined me immediately, but he could not feel anything with his trained surgeon's fingers. But I could! He examined my breast again the next morning and still couldn't feel any lumps. On the third day, he found something. By this time it felt enormous to me! My husband and I both believed it was a small cyst, but, even though 80% of breast lumps are benign, he suggested a mammogram just to be safe.

Several years ago I had taken advantage of an American Cancer Society screening program on mammography, so I already had a "normal" film on file. My lump did not visualize on the new mammogram. Usually this indicates a benign (non-cancerous) tumor, but I still wasn't satisfied and decided to get a biopsy, a surgical procedure where the tissue, in my case the offending lump, is removed and tested to determine what it is.

My biopsy came back POSITIVE! I had breast cancer! I had a potentially fatal disease. My whole life suddenly changed. I have a loving husband, two small children, and a wonderful exciting life. How could I have breast cancer? I thought that only happens to other people—the lady down the street or someone's auntie—BUT NEVER TO ME! So why me? The question, I learned, does not have a rational answer.

Following my surgery I learned a great many things about breast cancer. Most importantly, I learned that because I had practiced breast self-examination and had found the lump so early, I was going to get well. Less than half of breast cancers are found that early, but because of greater educational efforts, and especially BSE, the numbers are getting better and better.

Another important thing I learned is that mammography is not infallible. It is an important diagnostic aid but cannot replace self-examination.

I learned that no one knows the lumps and bumps in your breasts like you do. You alone can determine that you have a new one, or that one somehow feels different. The only way to keep up with these changes is with weekly examinations. In fact, ninety percent of breast cancers are discovered by women themselves. Self-examination is extremely important since a fast growing breast cancer doubles in size about every 28 days—not just gets larger, but DOUBLES! Once a tumor is large enough to be felt, it may have been growing for two years or more!

If your mother or sister has had breast cancer you are twice as likely to develop it. No one in my family has ever had breast cancer—so much for statistics. I spoke with lots and lots and lots of doctors about breast cancer and the one thing they all agreed on was that early detection means a higher cure rate. Breast self examination CAN make the difference. When you feel something that wasn't there before, or has changed in some way, go see your doctor immediately! To delay treatment could make you a statistic.

In 1979, it was estimated that 1 in 14 women would develop breast cancer; in 1982, the estimated rate was 1 in 11. Some statisticians estimate that by the year 2000 it will be 1 woman in 7 who develops breast cancer.

If you do not know the technique of breast self-examination, ask your doctor to show you. The American Cancer Society has endless free pamphlets, films and educational programs on breast cancer detection. Because a bi-yearly exam by your physician is not frequent enough, the responsibility of regular breast examination lies with each one of us. A weekly personal examination takes minutes and educates your fingers about your breasts so they will be able to detect any changes long before someone else might. There are many reasons other than cancer for that lump, but you will never know what it is until you see a doctor. You owe it to yourself and those that love you to check thoroughly and consistently for breast cancer. Because I found that tiny lump when I did and received immediate and appropriate treatment, I know I am going to live to see my two boys grow up. Remember 1 out of every 10 women will develop breast cancer—136,000 new cases in the U.S. this year. Learn to take care of yourself; no one else can do it for you. Breast cancer recognizes no favorites; if it can happen to me, it can happen to you!

Author's note: Since Carole wrote her article, many women have told me that they check their breasts on a more regular basis. Two of these women found an early cancer, had their surgery, and are doing well.

TESTICULAR CANCER

I should be "hardened" after so many years of seeing patients with cancer, but I'm not. I still cry right along with the family.

Several years ago, a good friend of mine, a young man of 35, called me and asked, "John, which doctor should I see? I've noticed a small lump in my left testicle for the last couple weeks." I advised him to see Dr. Haines (one of our urologists on Maui) immediately. He did, and the following day Dr. Haines and I removed his left testicle which contained a small, but very malignant, cancer. I cried when I told his wife what we had found because I felt the enormous threat to him, his wife and to their sons. After his surgery, he was referred to a Mainland cancer center which specializes in the treatment of testicular cancer. Fortunately, after additional surgery and months of chemotherapy, he now has almost a 100% chance of being cured of this cancer.

Cancer of the testicle accounts for only 1% of all cancers in males, but it is THE MOST COMMON CANCER IN MALES AGES 15 TO 35. On Maui we see only two or three cases a year, but that is more than enough. A young man or boy with this cancer is understandably devastated.

Once again cancer education is important, because the sooner the man discovers the tumor and reports it to his doctor, the better the chance for cure.

Most lumps and swellings in the scrotum are not cancer, but only your physician should make the diagnosis. Small cysts, hydroceles, hernias, and epididymitis (an infection) can all produce abnormal swellings. Sometimes a diagnosis is difficult and a biopsy will be necessary.

Early detection IS important, and so self-examination by males should be done every month. Just as physicians encourage women to examine their breasts frequently for early detection of breast cancer, testicular examination by a man is equally as important. The next time your teenage son or your husband is at the doctor's office, ask for an examination and instructions about self-examination.

There is no known cause for testicular cancer, but it is known that testicles which are undescended (not present in the scrotum) at birth have fourteen times the risk of developing cancer as do normal testes. Boys with undescended testicles should have them brought into the scrotum by surgery as early as possible.

Testicular cancer is rare but extremely dangerous. Early detection by boys and young men will increase the chances for cure.

LIP CANCER

Lip cancer is an uncommon cancer, but when it occurs it must be treated immediately to avoid disfigurement or possible death. There is   considerable discrimination with this cancer as the number of cases affecting men outweigh those affecting women 50 to 1. Another interesting statistic is that the lower lip is affected in 99% of the cases.

The major cause of this cancer is believed to be the sun's ultraviolet rays hitting the lower lip year after year. Typically it takes 50 or more years for the cancer to develop, but then watch out! Previously, women appeared to be protected because their occupations did not over-expose them to the sun, but I'm not sure that this is true any longer. Moreover, lipstick worn by women certainly blocks those dangerous rays. Another causative agent is believed to be a cold sore (herpes simplex) recurring on the same area of the lip.

Lip cancer will usually begin as a small nodule or ulcer on the lower lip. If the usual medicated creams and ointments do not quickly heal the ulcer, then a biopsy is indicated.

Like most cancers, the earlier the diagnosis, the better the chance for cure. If the lip cancer is less than one centimeter (1/2 inch) in size, then minor surgery is required, and the cure rate is 98%. When the cancer is greater than two centimeters (one inch), a more major operation is required. In addition, there is a greater risk that the cancer will spread to the lymph nodes of the neck. Then x-ray treatment or radical surgery is necessary, but even then the cancer may continue to spread. Obviously, the intelligent choice is to have the cancer treated at its earliest stage.

Ladies, take a good look at your husband's lower lip before he gives you that next kiss (I hope it won't be too long), and if you see a lump or a sore, get him to see his doctor before it is too late.

BREAST CANCER

BREAST CANCER. Those two words cause more fear in women than they should. Because they cause so much fear, many women refuse to examine their breasts, or do so in a rapid and incomplete manner. As a result, they try to find nothing and often miss an early tumor.

"Life," "cure" and "non-mutilation" are words that can be associated with breast cancer if a woman practices frequent breast examination. If she detects a cancer early (1/2 inch in size or smaller), not only does she stand a high probability of being cured, but with today's surgery she can possibly retain her breast or have reconstructive plastic surgery.

For seventy years the only surgery for breast cancer was the "radical mastectomy", in which the breast and chest muscles were removed. This procedure was necessary because, before cancer education, a woman would often wait to see her doctor until the tumor had grown to the size of an orange and had invaded the muscles. During the 1970's, with better cancer education, women were discovering their breast cancers earlier. Surgeons found that performing a "simple mastectomy", where the breast is removed and the chest muscles are left intact, gave equally good survival results.

In 1980, doctors from large cancer centers reported that when the cancer was small, one inch in diameter or less, an equal number of cures was obtained by widely excising the tumor and treating the remaining breast tissue with x-ray therapy. With this procedure most of the natural breast was retained. It was still necessary to do a small operation under the arm to remove some of the lymph nodes in order to determine if the tumor had spread. The earlier and smaller a cancer is found, the less often it will spread to the lymph nodes and to other parts of the body.

When it is necessary to remove the breast, reconstruction can be performed by a plastic surgeon. The area where the breast was removed is rebuilt to resemble the remaining breast. Usually a satisfactory result can be achieved.

Hopefully in the future there will be some form of immunization against breast cancer, but until that time early surgery is the only cure for this disease, and self-examination is imperative.

How often is it necessary to examine your breasts? Once a month is not enough. It would be too easy to forget to do your examination or to forget which lumps are normal and which are not. To protect your teeth you have learned to brush them twice a day. To protect your life you need to examine your breasts carefully once a week. Frequent breast examination can detect a cancer at a stage where a cure is probable and preservation of the breast is possible.

4 Infections

APPENDICITIS—
STILL A DANGEROUS ILLNESS

Last night I was called to the hospital to evaluate a young woman who had had abdominal pain for the previous twenty-four hours. I diagnosed a case of acute appendicitis, and an hour later she was asleep in the operating room. During surgery I removed an already ruptured appendix. Peritonitis (infection in the abdomen) had occurred, but with modern-day antibiotics and intravenous fluids she should survive this serious illness. This has not always been the case and I thought the reader might be interested in the history of appendicitis and the progression to the modern-day treatment.

Appendicitis has been known since antiquity. Even mummies in Egypt have been found with scarring in the right lower part of the abdomen, indicating appendicitis. In the 1700's, when autopsies were first utilized to discover the causes of death, a frequent finding was that of an abscess around a gangrenous appendix. For the next hundred years many medical authors wrote about this infection surrounding the cecum and appendix. Operations were usually confined to drainage of the abscess which would "point" at the skin; nevertheless, recovery was extremely rare once appendicitis occurred.

In the middle of the 19th century, with the advent of ether and chloroform anesthesia, more operations were performed but usually only as a "last resort", and frequently the patient would die from peritonitis. The cause of the abscess was not recognized until 1886 when Dr. Reginald Fitz described the progression of acute appendicitis to perforation, abscess formation, and peritonitis. He was the first physician to recommend early surgery when the first signs of appendicitis occurred rather than waiting for perforation.

From that time on, surgeons would operate earlier and earlier when the patient presented signs and symptoms of appendicitis. Frequently, as with my case last night, perforation and peritonitis had already occurred and, unless the individual was extremely strong, death would follow after a prolonged period of infection. This was the fate of Dr. Walter Reed, the famous Army Surgeon who had discovered the cause for yellow fever. In November 1902, he developed appendicitis and at surgery was found to have a perforation with peritonitis. After three-weeks of increasing infection, he died.

With the advent of antibiotics in the 1940's, and the "super antibiotics" of today, we are now able to control and cure peritonitis. Despite these advances, surgeons still prefer to operate early and remove the appendix before it ruptures.

The symptoms of appendicitis can frequently be tricky, especially since similar symptoms occur with many other illnesses. The patient begins with a mild "upset stomach" for several hours, followed by vomiting. (How many of us have had similar symptoms with intestinal flu?) The pain slowly switches to the lower right side of the abdomen. This area becomes quite tender when the patient or the doctor pushes on the skin. By this time the patient usually has developed a fever and the blood count has become elevated, indicating an infection. Sometimes the pain suddenly subsides (as was the case with my recent patient), only to recur and become more intense within the hour. When the pain disappears it is an indication that the appendix has ruptured. Then the bacteria spreads throughout the abdomen, and the return of increased pain is a sign of peritonitis. Hopefully, before this happens, the patient has seen a physician and treatment is already under way.

Appendicitis still remains a very common condition and we see about fifteen cases a month at our hospital. It is not an illness to be taken lightly. If you or someone in your family experience some of these early symptoms, an immediate visit to your doctor may prevent serious complications.

SHINGLES — YOU'LL NEVER FORGET THE PAIN

Shingles on your roof
Will keep you from the rain
Shingles on your back
Will only cause you pain

Ask any patient who has suffered the pain of shingles, and his eyes will probably water as he relates his experiences. Herpes zoster (shingles) is caused by the varicella-zoster virus which also causes chicken pox in children. After once infecting the body, the virus will lie dormant in one of the nerves for years before being reactivated and causing the symptoms of shingles.

During the first forty-eight hours a person with shingles experiences only pain. This can be very perplexing to the doctor. Frequently x-rays are taken of the chest, gallbladder or kidneys to look for the cause of this pain. After forty-eight hours the typical vesicles (blisters) break out along the path of a nerve, and the diagnosis becomes "painfully" obvious. The patient is usually relieved to know that it is not the gallbladder causing the trouble, but is not happy about the continuing burning pain.

Until a few years ago, nothing could be done to shorten the course or to relieve the pain of shingles. Now, a new drug named acylovir is effective against the virus. It can be given either as a pill or by injection, for the more serious cases. However, the infected area will be sensitive to touch and temperature for months to come.

Approximately 70% of the cases involve one of the trunk nerves running on the chest or abdomen. These are painful; but, the most debilitated patients are those who are unfortunate to have shingles affect one of the nerves of the face. These patients should be admitted to the hospital to be given pain shots and one of the new anti-virus drugs. The drugs vidarabine and acyclovir must be injected into a vein and may create serious side effects. The benefits must be weighed against those dangers.

If you are given a choice, take your shingles on your roof rather than on your back.

AIDS

What a difference six years makes! In September of 1983, I wrote an article on a newly discovered disease—AIDS. In only a few short years, most of the information in the article has become outdated. This is because AIDS has been the most intensely studied disease in the history of medicine, and a large amount of knowledge has been learned in a short period of time.

The 1983 article contains these statements: "The disease has no known cause or treatment; there have been 1,972 cases in the U.S., seven in Hawaii, and none on Maui; no cases of AIDS have been reported from routine blood transfusions; the disease is confined to homosexual males, intravenous drug abusers, Haitian entrants to the U.S., and hemophiliacs." We now know that all of these statements are false!

In a short period of time we have learned that the disease is caused by a retrovirus which attacks the T-helper cells in the body's immune system, leaving the body unable to fight off rare, but fatal, diseases. The virus has now been named the Human Immunosuppresive Virus (HIV). Soon after this discovery, researchers developed a blood test which can determine whether or not a person has been infected by the virus, even though the person displays no symptoms. They have also learned that the incubation period (time from exposure to onset of symptoms) may be 5 to 10 years! This makes the investigation and possible cure of the disease far more difficult than with other diseases.

From 1983 to 1989, HIV cases in the U.S. have increased from 1,972 to more than 37,000, and so far 21,000 of these individuals have died. During the same period, cases in Hawaii have increased from 8 to 165, and 88 of these have died.

The most frightening estimate, with the help of the AIDS blood test, is that between 1 to 1 1/2 million Americans have been infected with the virus. Only time will tell whether or not all of these individuals will develop the disease, spread it to others, or die.

Six years ago I reported that only homosexual males, intravenous drug users, Haitians and hemophiliacs were infected with the disease. The virus has now entered the heterosexual arena where partners pass the virus to each other. Equally important, there are now many cases where the husband has infected his wife, and the wife, their unborn child. A great concern is that the virus will be passed into the sexually active young population in high schools and colleges, and that it may be five to ten years before symptoms develop to alert physicians as to the magnitude of the problem.

Casual day-to-day contact, as a hand-shake or a hug, is not believed to be dangerous, but "small" accidents in hospitals have resulted in the rare infection of health professionals. This has caused a great fear among the doctors, nurses, lab technicians and other hospital personnel. An accidental "needle stick", after the needle had been used on an AIDS patient, may mean not only an end to one's career but to one's life! The Center for Disease Control (CDC) has recommended that hospital personnel wear gloves whenever handling "body fluids" of "any" patient. Unfortunately, no one has designed a glove which will prevent a needle stick and still allow a surgeon to have the necessary "feel" in order to perform an operation. As a result, several surgeons on the Mainland have refused to treat patients with AIDS. Their refusal is contrary to the oath doctors have taken to help their fellow man.

Six years ago no one was known to have contracted AIDS from receiving a blood transfusion, although hemophiliacs had become infected from extracts of blood. Now there have been numerous examples where patients who received blood for operations later developed AIDS or tested positive for HIV. All blood is now tested for the AIDS virus, but even a negative test does not guarantee that the blood is 100% safe. The blood donor may have acquired the infection so recently that his blood test is still negative, when actually his blood contains the virus. This fear has caused doctors to order blood transfusions only when the patient is facing a life-threatening condition.

There is no known cure for AIDS. Ninety-eight percent of patients will die within three years. Within the last several years a drug has been released by the Federal Drug Administration (FDA) which inhibits the multiplication of the virus within the body. The virus is not killed, only slowed down. Zidovudine (AZT) has many serious side effects, costs about $10,000 per year, and is the only option available for AIDS patients at present. Other drugs are being tested, but they will not be released until they are determined to be safe.

The hope for the future lies in the discovery of a vaccine which will protect a person from contracting this lethal disease. Several vaccines will be tested this next year, but it may be five to ten years before a vaccine is ready for use by the general public. Unfortunately, all those who are now infected, or who will become infected during the next ten years, will probably die from their disease. It is not surprising, then, that there is at present a heavy emphasis on protection and prevention rather than waiting and hoping for a cure.

A few years from now, when I write my next *"Update on AIDS,"* hopefully I can report better news and more advances in the battle against this killer. The best news would be a cure.

A LETTER TO SARA

Dear Sara,

Carole and I enjoyed your stay with us during your recent visit. The years have flown by, and we have watched you grow and mature from a high school student to a college graduate, and now a businesswoman on the Mainland. We love you as much as we do our own children, and it is because of this love that I want to continue the discussion we shared during your last evening on Maui.

I was surprised that you were not more "up-to-date" on the threat of AIDS! It is the single, greatest danger facing young people today. The Hawaii Department of Health recently reported that the AIDS virus is now carried by one out of every 200 people! It is not known how many of these people will die from AIDS, but the estimates are between 50% and 100%! Of enormous concern is that these people may not develop symptoms for several years (sometimes five or ten years) during which time they may infect many others. Month after month the reports about the numbers becoming infected get worse. No longer is is just the male homosexual. No longer is it just the drug user. Now the heterosexual has become infected and is rapidly passing along this killer.

Surprising as it seems, the AIDS virus does not kill. Instead, it weakens the body so that other diseases can attack it. The Human Immunosuppressive Virus (HIV) destroys the T-Helper cells in the body's immune system, and the weakened system is assaulted by strange sounding bacteria and tumors such as Pneumocystes caranii and Kaposi's sarcoma. They might not win the war on the first attack; however, as the body becomes weaker and weaker, they finally win.

About the only thing that is known for sure about AIDS is how it is spread and how it is NOT spread. The virus can be isolated from the different body fluids such as semen, tears, saliva, blood and vaginal secretions. It is spread most commonly through sexual intercourse, both anal and vaginal, contaminated needles from drug users, and the rare contaminated blood transfusion. At this time there have been no cases of AIDS developing from casual contact at work, school or home. Rare cases of AIDS have occurred in doctors and hospital personnel who have been contaminated by accidental needle sticks.

So if a young adult is not a drug user and doesn't need blood transfusions, how can one protect oneself from this certain death? SAFE SEX is how. The casual sex of the 1970's is dead, and so are many of the participants. If you have sex today, you will be exposing yourself not only to your partner, but also to his contacts from the PREVIOUS FIVE TO TEN YEARS!

Sex-after-marriage is the safest bet, providing the spouse has been celibate for at least five years; however, because many 20-year-olds (and those a good deal older) are sexually active, sex before marriage is still a prevalent activity. At the very least, a young adult should have known her/his potential sex-partner for a long time before engaging in relations. It is Russian roulette to have a sexual engagement with a stranger, and most of the gun's chambers are loaded!

The Surgeon General, Dr. C. Everett Koop, offers advice on extra protection for sexually active, unmarried young adults. He strongly advises that the male always use a condom for HIS protection and that the female insists that the male use one for HER protection. The young are apparently listening to him, because the sales of condoms have increased dramatically. Nonetheless, more education is necessary if this terrible disease is to be contained and eventually controlled. Researchers believe that it will be five to ten years before a vaccine is developed, but by then millions will have become infected or have died from AIDS.

Until the protection of a vaccine becomes available, parents must protect their children by educating them. I hope that the parents who read this letter will talk to their children. Education is the first line of defense. This is also why I am writing to you, Sara, and offering you this fatherly advice. Talk to your friends and warn them about the immeasurable danger AIDS poses for

those who are either careless or uneducated about sexual contact.
Sara, we want you to live.

Love,
John

PINKEYE

On Sunday we went whale-watching, and I made the mistake of not wearing my sunglasses. For hours I had to squint into the afternoon sun and the blowing Kona wind. On Monday morning my son, Noel, pointed at my right eye and uttered a tender, concerned statement, "Ick, your eye is bleeding." Indeed, the mirror revealed that I had a subconjunctival hemorrhage. I would have to explain my red eye to my patients over and over again the following week. A "red eye" has numerous causes other than the sun and wind, and a discussion can educate us all.

The white of the eye is the sclera, which is its protective outer coat. However, it is the conjunctiva, a thin, transparent membrane over the sclera that contains small blood vessels and becomes pink or red when injured. We all have had a fleck of dust in our eyes, and after rubbing the eye have had it turn pink. This happens because the blood vessels dilate to bring more blood to the eye to fight the injury or infection.

Inflammation of the conjunctiva is termed "conjunctivitis," and is the most common of all eye diseases. The causes of conjunctivitis can generally be divided into infectious, allergic, irritative and a large group of "other" causes. There are at least 50 different bacteria, viruses, parasites or other infectious agents which can give rise to conjunctivitis, but the one we hear the most about is "pink eye". The medical term for "pink eye" is acute catarrhal conjunctivitis and usually occurs as an epidemic. The most common causes are the bacteria pneumococcus and H. aegyptius, which will produce a very red eye and a moderate amount of mucopurulent (pus) drainage. Other bacteria, such as

H. influenza, E. coli, Proteus and S. aureus (staph) can cause less severe or chronic conjunctivitis. Any drainage of pus from your eye is a signal to see your physician immediately.

A year ago, Hawaii had a small epidemic of Acute Hemorrhagic Conjunctivitis, which was frightening to the victims. It is caused by an enterovirus (a special virus) and produces pain, photophobia (fear of the light), tearing and subconjuctival hemorrhage (bleeding under the conjuntiva). The virus is transmitted by close person-to-person contact. There is no known treatment but, fortunately, all victims recover in five to seven days.

Trachoma, which is an eye disease caused by Chlamydial bacteria, has been infecting mankind since the 27th century B.C. Today it affects over 400 million of the world's population. It causes scarring of the conjunctiva, then the cornea, and finally blindness. The absence of trachoma in the U.S. (except among American Indians) is a credit to our public health system.

Allergic reactions cause the largest numbers of mild conjunctivitis among the population. Pollens, grasses, animal dander, etc... can cause not only sneezing, but also runny, red eyes. Smoke, wind, volcano smoke and ultraviolet light are irritants and, likewise, can cause conjunctivitis. Severe coughing or sneezing may result in hemorrhage (bleeding) beneath the conjunctiva, and it will take one to two weeks to clear.

The final cause of conjunctivitis (which you won't find in a medical textbook), is the 11:00 PM United flight from Honolulu to San Francisco. They don't call it the Red-Eye Express for nothing!

5 General Information

PRESIDENTS' ILLNESSES

Ronald Reagan should be given an award for medical education of the American public. The news coverage of his injuries and illnesses has enlightened us about gunshot wounds of the chest, colon cancer, colonoscopy, colon polyps, skin cancer of the nose, and now prostate hypertrophy and surgery. The President of the United States has no privacy and that is how it should be. His health may affect his decisions on national or international problems, ultimately affecting millions of lives.

A review of past presidents' illnesses shows that they are affected with the same diseases as their electorate. President Eisenhower complained that he couldn't even have a bellyache in private, and he was afflicted with many health problems during his terms. In 1955 he suffered a heart attack but recovered completely. Then in 1956 he had an attack of ileitis of the small intestine which required surgery. Eisenhower had a slight stroke in 1957, and the country was worried as to who was running the shop.

President Carter had his problems with hemorrhoids, Johnson had gallbladder surgery (and showed his scar to the world) and Kennedy had chronic back pain and trouble with his adrenal glands.

Truman was a healthy, scrappy president and attributed his good health to a brisk walk every morning. Nixon's ailments included viral pneumonia, thrombophlebitis (blood clot in the leg), and Watergate (a politically fatal disease).

The most fascinating medical history involves Franklin D. Roosevelt who, despite being stricken by polio in 1921, went on to become our only four-term president. He led the country out of the depression of the 1930's and then inspired us during World War II. But did his health hinder his decisions at Yalta in February 1945, when the fate of Europe was being decided? FDR died April 12, 1945, and the country was told that he died from a stroke. But was it a stroke? Medical investigators now believe that FDR died from a melanoma cancer (the black mole cancer) which had spread throughout his body. A review of pictures of Roosevelt in 1932, 1936 and 1940 show an enlarging black mole over his left eyebrow. In a photograph in August 1944, the mole had been removed and a surgical scar was present. This photograph also reveals that the President had lost considerable weight. The American voters were "assured" by FDR's physician that the President was healthy, and he was elected to a fourth term in November 1944. The photographs of FDR at Yalta show a severely ill president—similar in appearance to the many terminal cancer patients I've seen. Did President Roosevelt die of metastatic melanoma? Did a terminally ill, mentally impaired president give away Europe at Yalta? The country may never know, particularly because FDR's medical records at Bethesda Naval Hospital disappeared after his death.

Former President Reagan should have received the "Medical Education Award of 1986." We were fortunate that he made such quick recoveries.

POLYPS IN THE COLON

Mushrooms in the colon? Ridiculous! The best description I can give of polyps (benign tumors) of the colon (the large intestine) is that the polyps look very similar to mushrooms. There is a large fleshy head hanging from a stalk attached to the inside wall of the large bowel.

Are these polyps dangerous and, if they are, what can be done about them? Most of the polyps remain benign (non-cancerous) during their lifetime, but many will change into a cancer. If not discovered in time, these "changed" polyps will kill their host.

Researchers now believe that all cancers of the colon originate from small or large polyps. If one could remove these polyps at an early stage it would be possible to prevent cancer of the colon! This is a very exciting possibility, since cancer of the colon is Hawaii's No. 1 form of cancer.

At the University of Minnesota, Dr. Gilbertson, through a 25-year study, proved the theory that cancers arise from the polyps. He removed all the polyps in the rectal area of 1,000 patients and followed up on each case annually. These patients had 85% fewer cancers of the rectal area than would be expected in a comparable 1,000 patients. Moreover, those cancers that did occur in that area were found and treated at such an early stage that all the patients survived their cancers.

How can these polyps of the colon be found before they become cancerous? It is usually the individual who notices that there has been blood with a bowel movement and reports this to his/her physician. As physicians, we have learned never to assume that the bleeding is from a "simple hemorrhoid." Your doctor must diligently rule out the possibility of an early cancer or polyp formation. The examination requires that the patient have a sigmoidoscopic examination and a barium enema.

Another way that polyps can be discovered at an early stage is through the stool guaiac test. This should be ordered routinely on individuals over the age of 45. With the help of the American Cancer Society, several screening programs have been offered here on Maui, and many polyps and early cancers have been discovered.

Once the polyp has been detected it can usually be removed without a major operation. Prior to the development of the colonoscope (an instrument that looks like a flexible small-caliber garden hose) a major operation at the hospital was necessary. This would have required general anesthesia, an incision into the abdomen, removal of part of the bowel, a hospitalization of at least a week, and patient recuperation (off work) for one to two months. The combined cost of the operation and hospitalization is about $7,000 and the patient would lose valuable time from work.

Now with the use of the colonoscope, most polyps can be removed without a major operation. The cost has been reduced to approximately $1000, and the patient is usually ready to return to work the following day.

Once the polyp is removed, the tissue is sent to the pathologist who determines if a cancer is present and whether or not there has been invasion (spread) of the cancer into the stalk (neck) of the polyp. Most polyps are not cancerous, but if a cancer is found, and there is no invasion, then no further surgery is necessary. If invasion is present, then an operation is necessary to remove that part of the bowel and the lymph nodes which may have trapped any cancer cells.

Early detection is the key to curing cancer of the colon. If you have noticed any blood in your bowel movement, please notify your physician immediately. If you are over the age of 45, request that your physician order a guaiac test as part of your next annual physical examination.

OSTEOPOROSIS

"Doctor, I'm getting shorter. Is there anything to worry about?" This is a common question from women who have passed the age of 50, and, yes, there is something to worry about. Osteoporosis (thinning of the bones) is common in women after their menopause, and it is due to the loss of calcium from the bones as the estrogen level begins to fall. Actually the ovaries begin to decrease the estrogen level while women are still in their 30's, but it is not until menopause that serious bone problems may develop.

It is believed that the hormone, estrogen, helps maintain the integrity of the strength of the bone by preventing the re-absorption (dissolving into the blood) of the calcium from the bone. When the calcium is lost, it is just like losing the cement from concrete—and the houses, or bones in this case, start to crumble.

Women past the age of 50 experience a marked increase in fractures of the wrist, hip and back. In fact, hip fractures are eight times more common in women than in men, partially because women live longer, but mainly because men's hip bones remain stronger. Men occasionally develop osteoporosis, but usually this is due to a lack of calcium from poor dietary habits.

In order to prevent these complications of hip and back fractures, can osteoporosis be detected early—and is there any treatment?

The first tip-off may be that a woman notices she has lost an inch or two in height since she was age 20. (Have the nurse measure your height the next time you are in your doctor's office.) Side-view x-rays of the chest give doctors a view of the vertebrae and help estimate the strength of the bones. Testing the blood for calcium content and enzymes is rarely helpful in detecting osteoporosis. New x-ray machines have been developed by NASA to detect osteoporosis in astronauts, and this test is now available at most hospitals.

Once a diagnosis of osteoporosis is made, medical treatment is advised in order to prevent further thinning of the bones and resultant fractures. There are four parts to the treatment, and each is equally important.

The first is an adequate intake of calcium. It has been determined that a daily intake of 1500 mgm of calcium is necessary as the estrogen level falls. This exceeds the calcium level in a normal diet, and women should see their physician or pharmacist for a calcium supplement.

In post-menopausal women, estrogens are essential to prevent further thinning of the bones. A small risk of cancer of the uterus occurs with women on long-term estrogens—but no increased risk of breast cancer. For a woman who has had a hysterectomy, there is no danger in taking long-term estrogens, but in the others it is recommended that the estrogens be cycled three weeks with a week of progesterone.

Exercise has been shown to retard bone loss and even to increase its strength. Tennis, running and exercise classes are important for as long as an individual can participate. In later years, walking has proved to be beneficial.

In 1982 a study at the Mayo Clinic showed that by adding sodium fluoride to the treatment (with calcium and estrogens) the fracture rate was reduced to under 10% of an untreated "control" group. Sodium fluoride appears to strengthen the bones much as it strengthens the teeth in children; however, not all patients were able to take the medicine because an irritation of the stomach and intestinal tract occurred in about half of the group.

While exercise, calcium, estrogen and fluoride may not be all the elements in the water at the fountain of youth for women, they will prevent osteoporosis and make their later years healthier and more enjoyable.

HIGH ALTITUDE ILLNESS

Having just returned from a wonderful vacation at Skyline Ranch located in the high mountains of Colorado, I want to share with you a bit of medical knowledge I acquired while away. If you plan to take a vacation to any location above an elevation of 10,000 feet, this information will be of particular interest.

The beauty of the snow-capped Colorado mountains with the meadows filled with columbine and aspen daisies was diminished the first two days of our family vacation because of rather severe headaches and some breathing difficulties. We were experiencing "acute high altitude illness" and a little preparation could have helped us avoid this discomfort.

Acute high altitude illness is the body's complex response to the decreasing pressure of oxygen in the air that you breathe at higher altitudes. The symptoms which develop may be as mild as headaches and lassitude, or very dangerous such as cerebral edema (swelling of the brain), pulmonary edema (excess fluid in the lungs), and retinal hemorrhages (bleeding in the back of the eyes).

The extent of discomfort or danger usually depends on several factors: the individual, as most people do not experience problems; the altitude, as reactions are not found below 8,000 feet and become more severe above 12,000 feet; and the amount of exercise the person is doing. The more strenuous the exercise the greater the risk of developing the illness.

Immediate treatment may be lifesaving and consists of quickly taking the patient to a lower elevation so that the body can re-equilibrate (normalize the body functions).

There are two methods of preventing acute high altitude illness and should be considered by anyone traveling to the "high country." First, spend a day at a location somewhat below 8,000 feet, allowing your body to adjust to a higher elevation. When you reach the next higher elevation, do not try to ski all the runs the first day and do not attempt to climb the mountain until the third day.

If you are still bothered by headaches and lassitude at high elevations, then, prior to your next trip, consider seeing your physician for a prescription for the drug acetazolamide (Diamox). This drug must be started before your departure and usually prevents the symptoms.

Last week, when my son, Noel, and I were standing on top of Mt. Wetterhorn (elevation 14,017 feet), I thought my elation and light-headedness was because of the beauty of the mountains which surrounded us. Perhaps I was only having a touch of high altitude illness.

HICCUPS, THEIR CAUSE AND CURE

How embarrassing! You've been invited to the boss's home for dinner and with your first bite of food—HICCUP! Everyone politely looks at you as though you are about to say something important. HICCUP! The second hiccup indicates to all that the siege is on, and the helpful suggestions begin. "Breathe into a paper bag." This slows the hiccups but doesn't stop them. HIC-CUP! "BOO!" Frightening you doesn't help. HICCUP! "Swallow this teaspoonful of sugar." Seconds tick by. Then silence. A cure has been found. After apologies, everyone turns his attention to dinner again. What happens when you have the hiccups? What can you do about them? Are they ever dangerous?

A hiccup is a primitive reflex, much like coughing, yawning or vomiting. Being associated with eating, it may have developed in order to dislodge food stuck in the esophagus (the tube from the mouth to the stomach). During hiccups there are intermittent, spasmodic contractions of the diaphragm (the muscle which helps you breathe) followed within 35 milliseconds by closure of the vocal cords. These two actions combined produce the body-shaking HICCUP — HICCUP — HICCUP!

Fortunately, the cure is not worse than the disease. Breathing into a bag or being "scared" rarely works, but slowly drinking cold water or swallowing a teaspoonful of granulated sugar will stimulate the nerve fibers in the esophagus, usually "break" the reflex, and stop the hiccups. If the hiccups are persistent, lasting for several hours, you should see your physician or go to a hospital emergency room. Several drugs (chlorpromazine, meto-clopramide) injected into the vein will usually cure the hiccups.

Ninety-nine percent of people with hiccups will have a benign course. Rarely do hiccups indicate a more serious disease. Brain tumors, meningitis, head trauma, tumors or diseases of the chest or upper abdomen can all produce hiccups, but usually there are many other symptoms to suggest the cause.

Embarrassing, maddening, frustrating—hiccups are all of these. At the next dinner party, if it is your boss who suddenly goes "HICCUP," your job may depend on how sympathetic and helpful you are.

HYPERVENTILATION

My grandmother used to say, "Too much of a good thing is bad for you." I never realized that she could have been talking about BREATHING! When an individual breathes too rapidly, he is diagnosed as having hyperventilation (hyper–excessive, ventilation –breathing). It is distressing and sometimes dangerous.

One of our natural survival reflexes is the production of adrenalin by the adrenal glands in response to stress. This is called the "fight or flight" reflex, as it prepares the body to either defend itself or to run away as quickly as possible. The adrenalin speeds up our breathing, increases the heart rate and dilates the blood vessels in our muscles to give them more blood and oxygen.

For the short term this is an important natural reflex, but if it becomes a chronic response to mild stress it can produce hyperventilation and all of its unpleasant side effects.

During the Civil War, military physicians treated many soldiers who complained of breathlessness, dizziness, pronounced fatigue, numbness of hands and mouth, and chest pain. Despite these complaints, no cause could be found. They named this condition "soldier's heart." We now call it "Hyperventilation Syndrome."

It is usually a self-perpetuating condition because as the patient experiences the symptoms, such as spasms of the hands, the more worried he becomes and the more rapidly he breathes. In turn, this produces more symptoms.

The time honored emergency room treatment is to have the patient breathe into a small paper bag until the symptoms clear. This procedure helps to increase the CO_2 in the lungs and blood stream and reverse the respiratory alkalosis which was the original cause of the hyperventilation symptoms.

The list of symptoms is long and includes weakness, fatigue, blurred vision, anxiety, depression, tingling around the mouth, hands and feet, lightheadedness, dizziness, fainting, headaches, palpitations, chest pain, difficulty taking a deep breath, and muscular cramps. No wonder a patient becomes frightened!

What can be done to help the patient deal with hyperventilation? First, the physician must exclude other illnesses that might be causing the same symptoms or be responsible for the reflex of increased breathing. Angina or other heart problems are high on the list. Next, the patient and family should be trained to recognize the symptoms so that they can break the hyperventilation cycle early by having the patient breathe into a paper bag. In addition, a group of drugs known as "beta-blockers" are effective in blocking the adrenalin response to mild stress. These drugs are frequently used by public speakers and actors/actresses to prevent symptoms of hyperventilation from occurring. There is also long-term treatment which requires behavior modification and relaxation therapy by a trained psychiatrist or psychologist.

Patients are surprised when they learn that something as simple as breathing too rapidly can cause such distressing symptoms. Don't throw away your lunch bag; you never know when you might need it!

CHEST PAIN

Fortunately not all chest pains are heart attacks or pneumonias, but some are. Knowledge of important signs and symptoms might save your life in the future.

Myocardial infarction (heart attack) is the most feared cause of chest pain and with good reason! The pain is usually described by the patient as being "tight" or "heavy," and is located behind the sternum (the bone in the center of the chest). It might be only a mild pain that lasts for several hours or it might be "crushing," followed by the collapse of the patient and death. Frequently a pain is also felt in the left arm or at the base of the neck. If you have this type of pain and it lasts for more than a few minutes, an immediate call to your doctor or the emergency room may save your life.

A similar type of pain that occurs during exercise and clears with rest is called anginal pain. This pain is also serious because it indicates that not enough blood and oxygen are getting to the heart muscle to supply its needs. Again—contact your doctor.

The pain of pneumonia (an infection in the lung) or of pleurisy (an infection of the lining of the lung) can be located anywhere in the chest and usually is made worse by taking a deep breath. Shortness of breath, fever and chest pain are the symptoms that usually cause a patient to seek medical help.

Shortness of breath and chest pain in a young adult can be symptoms of a pneumothorax (a collapsed lung). This occurs spontaneously or after exercise and is caused by a rupture of a blister on the surface of the lung. Immediate medical attention is necessary.

Many chest pains are caused by muscle strains, myositis (a cold in the muscle), or condritis (an irritation of the end of a rib). Heat, aspirin and rest usually provide relief.

"Heartburn" is a sign of a hiatal hernia (part of the stomach pushing up through the diaphragm) and is usually relieved by use of antacids such as Riopan. Visit your doctor to confirm the diagnosis and to obtain the proper medications to control the symptoms.

Problems in the abdomen can even refer pain up into the chest. Gallbladder attacks frequently cause pain in the back of the chest on the right side. Injuries to the spleen can produce pain in the left shoulder.

There are many more but less common causes of chest pain, such as aneurysms, shingles and ruptured discs in the back; however, these are for your doctor to determine.

I cannot stress too strongly the importance that adults seek immediate medical care for any central chest pain that lasts more than a few minutes. Your life could depend on it.

PAIN IN THE OKOLE

All that hurts around the okole is not hemorrhoids, so let's talk about some of the conditions that can cause pain in that "unmentionable" area. For those of you who are not familiar with the Hawaiian term OKOLE, it is the area of the body that you sit on.

The first and foremost cause of pain is from hemorrhoids, which are actually dilated or distended veins. "Internal" hemorrhoids (from the internal veins around the rectum) usually cause bleeding but rarely cause pain. It is the "external" hemorrhoids which develop the clots of blood that become extremely painful. These patients are never sitting when I see them in the examining room. It is too painful! But with minor surgery to remove the hemorrhoid, relief is obtained quickly, and the patient can resume normal activities.

Another painful condition of the okole is an anal fissure. This is a tear of the skin of the anal canal. The tear exposes the nerves of the area and, with each bowel movement, pain, spasms, and further tearing occurs. Frequently, surgery under anesthesia is required to correct this problem.

An abscess can develop about the rectum and cause fever and severe pain. The abscess must be incised and drained to provide relief and prevent further complications. One complication is the occurrence of a fistula, which is a tract or tube from the inside of the rectum to the outside skin. Although the fistula is not painful, it does cause repeated soiling of the underwear and recurrent infections.

Pilonidal sinuses and abscesses are located at the lower end of the spine and can be confused with the problems around the okole. "Pilo" comes from the Latin word meaning "hair," which is the cause of the problem of pilonidal sinuses and abscesses. You have probably noticed that babies will occasionally have little pukas (holes) in the skin over the lower end of the spine. As the child grows older and reaches adulthood, the hair that grows in this area can grow down into these pukas and form "hair balls" which finally become infected and progress to an abscess. For immediate relief the abscess must be incised and drained, but follow-up surgery is necessary to prevent recurrence.

Although taxes, neighbors, and government might be "pains in the okole," there are medical conditions of the rectum which will require a trip to your doctor.

LYMPH NODES – ALIAS PAC-MEN

Last week I was explaining the value of lymph nodes in the body to my young son, Nathan. I told him how the bacteria are trapped in the lymph nodes so that the lymphocytes can "gobble them up." Nathan's reply was that the lymph nodes were the PAC-MEN of the body. After regaining my composure, I told him that he was right.

The lymphatic system consists of small lymph vessels and hundreds of lymph nodes scattered in every conceivable place throughout the body. Most people know of the lymph nodes in the neck, which become swollen during a strep throat infection. Similar lymph nodes are present in the tissue under the skin, in the abdomen, surrounding the intestines, liver and stomach, and in the chest around the heart and lungs.

The function of the lymphatic system is to trap things that do not belong in the body, such as bacteria or cancer cells. Then the lymphatic system forms antibodies, the special proteins that attempt to destroy the bacteria or virus. (Thus far they have been unable to destroy the cancer cells.)

When a person develops a strep throat the lymph glands on either side of the neck become swollen as the bacteria are trapped and the body tries to "fight off" the infection. Prior to the use of modern antibiotics this was the body's only defense against infection. If our body and its lymphatic system were not strong enough, we would succumb to whichever bacteria or virus attacked us, whether it was polio, typhoid, streptococcus or one of a hundred other diseases.

The largest lymph node in the body is the spleen, a fist-sized organ in the abdomen snuggled up under the left ribs. The spleen, although more important in primitive animals, is still important in the human because it is a major source of antibody formation. Unfortunately, the spleen is frequently injured in accidents, but every effort is made to repair it so that future infections can be "gobbled up." This is an extremely important organ in young children since they are more susceptible to infections.

I wish that the lymphatic system was always our ally, but like every other part of the body it can undergo cancerous changes and threaten our lives.

Cancers which develop within the lymphatic system are called lymphomas. The most common one is Hodgkin's disease, which is usually seen in young adults. Fortunately, within the last 20 years great strides have been made in lymphoma treatment, and now 75% of victims can be cured with x-ray and chemotherapy (special drugs used to fight cancer).

Those small lumps in your neck and under your arms are really needed friends which fight infection; however, if they start to enlarge or become tender, see your physician to determine that you are not developing a serious problem.

ULCERS

"Oh, my ulcer is killing me!" This is a common refrain which has some degree of truth because ulcers can cause death.

What is an ulcer? It is a hole in the mucosa (the inside skin) of the stomach or the duodenum (the part of the small bowel just below the stomach). The hole can be as small as a pinhead or as large as a half-dollar; it can be shallow or can penetrate through the entire wall of the stomach.

"You give me an ulcer!" This can be true, but this "you" must include work, financial worries, the boss, your husband, wife or in-laws. Not to be excluded in "you" should be smoking, coffee, alcohol, aspirin and many other drugs. All of these "yous" increase the production of stomach acid, which can burn a hole (an ulcer) in the stomach or the duodenum.

Doctors know that increased acid causes ulcers in the duodenum, but they are less sure about why they form in the stomach itself. Three generally understood causes are regurgitation of bile, decreased resistance of the lining of the stomach, and cancer.

Cancer occurs in about ten percent of ulcers of the stomach, but it is extremely rare in ulcers of the duodenum. Physicians do not believe that benign (non-cancerous) ulcers become cancerous; however, as a cancer in the stomach grows, it may produce an ulcer in its center. With stomach ulcers it becomes essential to establish an accurate diagnosis as quickly as possible.

Analysis is now possible with the use of an instrument called a fiberoptic gastroscope. With this instrument the physician can look directly at the ulcer and take biopsies (small bites of the ulcer) to determine whether or not it is a cancer. This procedure takes about thirty minutes, either in the doctor's office or the outpatient department at the hospital.

Once the ulcer has been determined to be benign, or if the ulcer is in the duodenum, follow-up treatment is standard, but with a new twist. Diet is not as important as doctors once believed. For cxample, milk is now thought to produce more acid than it neutralizes. The ulcer patient should definitely stop smoking, avoid aspirin and refrain from alcohol.

Antacids like Gelusil, Maalox and Rolaids are helpful in neutralizing the stomach acid after it is produced. The new heroes in healing ulcers, however, are cimetidine (Tagamet) and ranitidine (Zantac). These drugs were developed in Europe and, after extensive investigation by the Federal Drug Administration, were released for use in the U.S.A. They work by blocking the production of stomach acid so that the ulcer can heal. The dosage is then maintained at a lower level to prevent the ulcer from recurring. The effectiveness of these drugs is proved by the 90% decrease in the number of operations now being performed for ulcers. In spite of this fact, over a period of time some patients will become resistant to the medications and surgery may be necessary.

The next time you have a persistent stomach pain, get a checkup by your physician. There's no sense in having an ulcer "kill you!"

DIVERTICULOSIS

The older we get the more we hear about diverticulosis and diverticulitis of the bowel. These are hardly household words, and I thought you might like to understand your doctor when, after your barium enema, he tells you, "Mr. or Mrs. Maui, you have diverticulosis." Instead of responding with a blank look, you can reply, "Well, I guess that means I must eat more roughage, and be sure that the rest of my family increases the amount of fiber in their diet."

The colon (the large bowel) is the intestinal area most frequently affected by diverticulosis. The colon starts on the lower right side of the abdomen (same area as the appendix), ascends up under your right ribs across to the left side of the abdomen, and down to the rectum. Its purpose is to reabsorb the liquids in our intestinal contents and act as an area of storage of the fecal contents prior to their elimination. Although the colon performs important functions, it is possible to live a healthy life without one. When the colon is removed, patients require an ileostomy appliance, a bag attached to the skin to catch the liquid.

Diverticulosis of the colon is the condition which occurs when the colon has developed numerous diverticula. What are diverticula? In trying to explain this condition to my patients, I use the comparison of a blowout developing on a tire. As the tire becomes weaker in one area it starts to bulge. As the bulge becomes larger, the tire becomes thinner until it finally ruptures or "blows out."

Essentially, that's what happens with the large bowel or colon. As the years go by and we continue to have constipated stools and "bear down" during our bowel movements, we increase the pressure inside the bowel. The mucosa, or inner lining of the bowel, is forced out through a weakened area in the bowel wall and a diverticulum is formed. After a while the colon looks like it has many "Mickey Mouse ears." Indeed, there may be as many as a hundred diverticula from one end of the large bowel to the other.

Other than having a strange appearance on a barium enema x-ray, is there any reason to worry about these diverticula? Most of the time they will behave themselves and not cause the patient any trouble. On the other hand, a common problem is an infection within the diverticulum called diverticulitis. The diverticulum becomes plugged with fecal material or stool, which contains numerous bacteria. The bacteria pass through the lining of the diverticulum into the surrounding tissue and cause an infection much like appendicitis. The patient will then develop tenderness in the area of the diverticulitis and become feverish. If a blood test shows evidence of an infection, then antibiotics must be started promptly. If the diverticulitis goes untreated it may develop an abscess or perforate and become as serious as a ruptured appendix.

Another complication of diverticulosis is serious bleeding. Occasionally, a diverticulum, one of the "Mickey Mouse ears," will have an artery on its inner lining rupture. Serious bleeding will occur and require transfusions or possibly surgery to remove most of the large bowel.

What causes these terrible problems in the bowel, and is there any way to cure or prevent them? Dr. Burkett, a famous British surgeon, has studied many civilizations whose diets have not become "modernized" (use of highly refined foods) and where people still eat large amounts of vegetable fiber and roughage. In these cultures, diverticulosis and diverticulitis are unknown. Moreover, appendicitis and cancer of the colon are rare.

Dr. Burkett and many other investigators recommend that we change our dietary habits and include more roughage, such as bran, whole grain cereals, whole grain breads, and an increased amount of fresh vegetables. I strongly recommend that parents develop eating habits in their children which include these dietary requirements.

For those of us who have already developed diverticulosis, is there any cure for this condition of the bowel? Unfortunately, the answer is no. The damage has been done. Contrarily, we know that if patients with diverticulosis maintain a high roughage diet, they will have fewer complications and more regular bowel functions.

GALLBLADDER PROBLEMS

After that delicious, greasy dinner last night of Portuguese soup, pork chops, mashed potatoes and gravy, I am waiting for the telltale symptoms of gallbladder disease. It is signaled by pain up and under my right ribs, nausea, and vomiting, followed by a trip to the emergency room! Fortune has smiled on me, however, and I have escaped this time.

Gallstones and their complications constitute the fourth most frequent cause for hospitalization among adults and will affect 20-30% of us during our lifetime. Since surgery of the gallbladder for gallstones or for cholecystitis (infection of the gallbladder) remains one of the most common operations among American adults, the public needs to be well informed about gallbladder disease and what can be done about it.

There have been many scientific investigations into the causes of this disease during the past 100 years. We now believe that gallstones form because of stasis, or failure of the bile to empty from the gallbladder. The cause of this stasis is unknown and may be related to either a lack of contraction of the gallbladder or to anatomical variations.

Once gallstones appear, 20-25% of the patients will develop an inflammation of the gallbladder, which can be as serious as appendicitis. Ten percent of these patients may die if the gallbladder ruptures from the infection.

The gallbladder itself does not serve a vital function in human beings and acts only as a storage sac for the bile, which is produced by the liver. There is concentration of the bile while it is held in the gallbladder. After ingestion of a fatty meal, the gallbladder will contract, emptying the bile into the intestine which then assists in the digestion of fatty foods.

A person who has had the gallbladder removed will have perfectly normal digestion as the bile from the liver, rather than being stored in the gallbladder, is emptied directly into the intestine.

The symptoms of gallstones range from none at all—many people live their entire lives in harmony with their gallstones—to the other extreme of severe pain, infection, perforation and death. The first sign of problems with gallstones is usually pain on the right side of the abdomen just beneath the ribs. Sometimes the pain penetrates through to the back or to the lower right chest. Frequently this attack will occur following a "fatty" meal. I can remember my father awakening many times at night complaining of "rotten food" that he had eaten at a restaurant. Actually it was his gallbladder acting up, which he didn't discover until ten years later. The reason for this pain is that the gallbladder is contracting and trying to squeeze the gallstones out through the small duct (or tube) that drains from the gallbladder.

Sometimes the gallbladder is successful and squeezes a stone down into the common duct, and another set of symptoms develops. When the common duct is blocked the bile cannot drain from the liver to the intestine. After a period of several days the patient will become jaundiced (yellow), although the pain itself may have subsided.

The increasing jaundice is dangerous to the liver since a high level of bile in the blood can cause cirrhosis. This is scarring in the liver which may cause the liver to fail and result in death.

During surgery it becomes important not only to remove the gallbladder and its gallstones, but also to remove the gallstone within the common duct so that bile can drain unobstructed into the intestine.

The other major reason for removing the gallbladder with gallstones is that 25-50% of these gallbladders will ultimately develop acute cholecystitis, an infection in the gallbladder. This not only causes pain but results in a high fever, elevated blood count, perforation, and possibly death.

Rather than waiting until the infection occurs, most surgeons have found it safer and easier to do surgery during periods when the patient first experiences pain from the gallstones. This is why most physicians recommend the elective removal of the gallbladder if gallstones are found on x-ray.

The final complication of gallstones is the rare but definite risk of cancer developing in the gallbladder from the chronic irritation of the gallstones.

Next week, when my wife, Carole, and I are at Ann Ferguson's house and Ann serves us her delicious Portuguese soup, I'll limit myself to one serving in the hope of avoiding a gallbladder attack.

INGUINAL HERNIA

"What? Why? How? What is a hernia? Why should I worry about it? How do I get it fixed?" These are the questions patients ask about hernias. A hernia is a protrusion of any tissue (intestine, fat, lung, etc...) into an area where it doesn't belong. There are many types of hernias such as an umbilical (belly button) hernia, hiatal hernia (where part of the stomach squeezes into the chest), internal, diaphragmatic and other hernias. Because the inguinal (groin) hernia is the most common, I want to focus on it in some detail.

Inguinal or groin hernias can be divided into direct and indirect types. In the direct variety, the bulge protrudes straight out and results from a splitting of the fascia (the fibers of the abdominal wall). This usually occurs in older individuals since the strength of the fascia tends to break down with age. The indirect inguinal hernia can occur as a combination of a congenital hernia sac (a sac the patient was born with) and an event, such as lifting a heavy object. However, the patient frequently does not remember the "event" after noticing the bulge.

The congenital sac is present in all of us during our embryonic months, but it usually closes or obliterates itself before birth in 90% of cases. Fortunately not all of the other 10% will develop a hernia, but the stage is set. Then with an episode of lifting, severe coughing or other abdominal straining, a loop of intestine pushes its way into the sac, past the internal ring (a muscular ring to hold the intestines where they belong) and a "bulge" is born—the first sign of a hernia.

The patient can push on the bulge and sometimes the intestine will "squish" back into the abdomen. But once the bulge or hernia has started, it will recur, getting larger as the months and years pass.

Why should you worry about it? In addition to the discomfort of a hernia, there is a definite danger in delaying its repair. Occasionally, when the intestine squeezes into the hernia sac, it becomes incarcerated (gets trapped) and cannot be pushed back into the abdomen. The longer the intestine stays in the sac, the more edematous (swollen) it becomes. Finally the swelling becomes so great that the blood cannot get through the ring to nourish the intestinal loop, and it dies. Without immediate surgery, the patient will develop shock and ultimately die. In order to prevent this tragic sequence, physicians recommend the routine repair of hernias unless there are other more serious medical problems.

The usual surgical procedure for a hernia repair takes about one hour and consists of excising (cutting out) the congenital sac, strengthening the weakened fibers with sutures or a patch, and closing the internal ring.

Most hernia operations are performed in surgi-centers and the patient goes home the afternoon of the surgery. The chance of a hernia recurring following a repair is only two percent.

All things considered, if you have a hernia I would advise you to have it repaired.

6 INJURIES

THE TRAUMA TEAM

I enjoyed watching the NFL Monday night football game when the Chicago Bears whipped the New York Giants 34 to 19. The Bears' quarterback, Mike Tomczak, played a sensational game as he led his team to victory. The real victory, however, resulted from a TEAM effort: Tomczak could not have been successful without his great receivers, fullbacks, offensive linemen and defensive team. The same is true for a surgeon. Trauma surgery could not be successful without a team effort.

Saturday morning, at about 2:30 AM, Suzie (not her real name) fell asleep while driving her car and ran into a tree. She demolished her car and received extensive injuries. The first members of the medical team to reach the accident were the ambulance crew, C.S. Zibiack and Trish Morine, who carefully removed Suzie from the wreck, protecting her neck and back and splinting her legs for transportation.

On arrival at the Emergency Room, Dr. Allen Spain, the ER physician, quickly evaluated Suzie's condition. IV's, blood studies and x-rays were started. He also phoned me because I was the trauma surgeon on call that night. At 3:00 AM I was on my way.

When I arrived in the ER, Allen was passing an endotracheal tube into Suzie's trachea (the wind-pipe going to the lungs). She had sustained many fractures of her facial bones and with the extensive bleeding she was actually drowning in her own blood. As Dr. Spain skillfully inserted the tube, Suzie's breathing improved immediately.

With patients who have multiple injuries, the general surgeon is called "to quarterback" the team. He must evaluate all the injuries, call the other specialists, determine which injuries must be treated first and often perform life-saving operations on the abdomen, chest or blood vessels.

Suzie's most immediate problem was the fractures of the facial bones, and Dr. Spain had called Dr. Andrew Don, an ear-nose-throat specialist, who arrived within minutes. With the endotracheal (breathing) tube in place, her fractures were no longer life threatening.

At this point I was most concerned as to whether or not she might have injured her spleen or liver, which can cause bleeding into the abdomen. For this reason, the next physician and team players to be called in (at 4:00 AM) were Dr. Gene Wasson, a radiologist, and the CT technician. I requested one CAT scan of Suzie's abdomen to look for blood or organ injury and another CAT scan of her brain to determine whether bleeding into the brain had occurred. Fortunately for Suzie, both of these examinations were negative. Suzie's next stop in preparation for surgery was the ICU (Intensive Care Unit).

Two other major injuries Suzie had received were deep lacerations into both knee joints. Dr. Robert Harvey, an orthopedic surgeon, repaired these later.

Dr. Don had detected bleeding from both ears, indicating a fracture at the base of the skull, and blood within her left eye. Further consultations were obtained from Dr. Roger Slater, a neurosurgeon, and Dr. William Perryman, an ophthamologist. The skull fracture would require no surgery, and the bleeding in the eye would clear with time.

Later that Saturday morning, Suzie underwent surgery. The anesthesia was administered by Dr. Billie Strothers. While Dr. Harvey repaired the lacerations of the knees, Dr. Don performed a tracheostomy (inserting a breathing tube into the neck), wired her broken facial bones together, and straightened her broken nose. The OR nurses were working overtime again that Saturday morning.

Once back in the ICU, the care of her respirator was supervised by Dr. Mark Hoskinson, an internist, and the respiratory therapists. The marvelous ICU nurses maintained a constant watch over Suzie while we all waited to see if she would awaken from her head injuries.

By Sunday morning she began to nod her head in response to questions. Monday found her fighting at her restraints and pulling at her tubes. She was unable to talk because her teeth were wired together and she was breathing through the tracheostomy in her throat. By Tuesday none of these obstacles was stopping Suzie!

The ICU provides a board with large letters printed on it, so that when patients cannot talk, they can spell out words by pointing to the letters. When I made my rounds Tuesday morning, Suzie was spelling out every question she could think of. "What happened?" "How long will I be here?" "Will I be able to walk again?" "Was anyone else in the car?" After we had answered all her questions, she spelled out two more words. First she pointed to me and to the nurses and then, pointing to the letters, spelled out, T-H-A-N-K Y-O-U.

Our team will never go to the Super Bowl, but this was a super victory.

HOW SHOULD YOU TREAT A SPRAIN?

HOT OR COLD? Heat or ice? Which treatment should people use for a twisted ankle? Yesterday, one of my patients said, "I knew that I should apply one or the other, so I flipped a coin and soaked my twisted ankle in warm water." I replied, "You lost the flip." Successful use of heat or ice demands a knowledge of the effects of temperatures on the body. Heat applications cause the tissue to have increased enzyme activity, oxygen demand, inflammation response, capillary permeability (with resultant tissue swelling), and dilation of the blood vessels. Heat also increases tendon flexibility and muscle contractility while decreasing the viscosity (thickness) of joint fluids; it also increases nerve conduction. Cold applications have the opposite effect of all of the above, with the major benefits of decreased oxygen demand, inflammation response, nerve conduction, tissue swelling and constriction of the blood vessels.

Cold applications will gradually provide deep penetration into the tissues, while most hot applications will only affect the superficial layers as the dilated blood vessels quickly carry away the heat. As a result, an effective way of delivering heat deep into the tissues rests on using ultrasound.

So how can this information be used in treatment? Acute injuries, such as sprained ankles, pulled muscles, burns and bruises, will heal more quickly if the swelling and inflammation are kept to a minimum, and this can only be achieved by cold application. Cold treatments also decrease nerve conduction, which the body interprets as less pain. Since most injuries result in maximum swelling during the first 48 hours, it is important to use cold applications immediately and then for 30 minutes every three to four hours. This should be continued for the first two days but longer times may prove necessary.

With chronic conditions, such as arthritis, backaches, sore muscles and stiff joints, heat is required because it will thin the joint fluids, relax the tendons and muscles and relieve pain (psychologically by making it feel better). Heat's draw back is that it accelerates inflammation (swelling) which is not good for any of these conditions. Moreover one MUST be more careful in applying heat than cold because a hot water bottle or a heating pad can cause a burn to the skin within a very short period of time. Extreme care MUST be used with older people for two reasons: their skin sensation might be impaired and their skin is very fragile.

So the next time you twist your ankle, wrap it in ice, elevate it on the end of the sofa, put some ice in a glass (for a soda of course), lay back and enjoy your favorite TV programs for the next two days.

TETANUS

"Ouch! That blankety-blank rusty nail! Now what am I supposed to do?"

Several times a week I have patients come into my office for minor abrasions or puncture wounds from nails or other sharp objects. Some of these patients could have easily treated themselves at home if they had known what to do. Others, who treat themselves, may allow an infection to occur and would be better off had they seen a doctor in the first place.

So what are you supposed to do if you have a minor abrasion or puncture wound? Everyone worries about tetanus or "lock jaw," and this is the usual reason that patients come to the office seeking a "tetanus shot."

Tetanus is a very serious infection. It may result in convulsions and death. Fortunately, tetanus is rare in this day of proper immunizations, and usually a physician will not see a case in his entire medical career. Only 100 cases of tetanus occur in the U.S. each year, and all occur among the poor who had not received immunizations as children.

Proper childhood "shots" include immunizations against diphtheria, pertussis (whooping cough) and tetanus. Four doses are given during the first year and a fifth dose at four to six years of age. This will give a relatively lifetime protection against these diseases. However, if a person sustains a contaminated cut or serious injury, a tetanus toxoid booster is recommended if he has not had one in the previous five years. This will increase his natural antibodies and protect him against this dreaded disease.

So which abrasions can a person take care of himself, and which ones require a visit to the doctor? A minor abrasion or scratch can be treated at home by washing it with soap and water and then applying Betadine or Silvadene ointment daily (ask your doctor for one of these to have at home for an emergency.) If the person has not had a tetanus booster within the last five years, then he should report to the doctor's office for the shot. If redness develops around a minor abrasion during the next several days, then the individual should see a physician, as an infection may be developing.

There are some "minor" injuries which should be seen by a physician as soon as possible. These are injuries to the hand and injuries to the lower legs or feet in the elderly or diabetic individual. Physicians do not want even minor infections to develop in the hands and, because of the poor blood supply in the elderly and the diabetic, a minor abrasion can progress and become either a severe infection or a deep skin ulcer.

My best advice is to check your children's and your own medical records to make sure that you have the protection provided by an—ouch—tetanus shot.

BEE STINGS

My family and I just returned from another wonderful vacation at Skyline Ranch near Telluride, Colorado. The fishing, horseback riding, mountain climbing, and renewing of old friendships were marvelous. The high mountain meadows were filled with wildflowers—columbine, larkspur, Indian paintbrush, aspen daisies—and bees. Unfortunately, there was an over-abundance of bees this summer and most guests were stung at least once. Reactions to the bee stings ranged from a minimal short irritation to an anaphylactic (life-threatening) reaction wherein one child almost died. Because bees and hornets are also common on Maui, a discussion of "what to do if you are stung" might be helpful to you in the future.

The stinging insects belong to the order Hymenoptera and include honeybees, bumblebees, yellow jackets, hornets and wasps. Most stings are from honeybees. Another ominous fact is that about 40 deaths a year occur from bee stings.

Most adults and children, once stung, will experience moderate pain in the area, a small elevated wheal of skin, a small amount of redness around the wheal and a moderate amount of itching near the sting. I experienced this annoying, but not dangerous, type of reaction after being stung. This mild reaction can be relieved by applying ice to the area.

Systemic or generalized reactions occur in less than one percent of stings. These reactions include "non-life-threatening" symptoms of generalized urticaria (welts on the arms, legs, chest and back), severe itching and swelling about the eyes, lips and ears. The more serious symptoms are laryngeal edema (tickle in the throat, gagging, difficulty swallowing, or voice change), bronchospasm (chest tightness or wheezing) and syncope (fainting). One of the teenage boys at the ranch experienced these symptoms but they were relieved by a 50 mg pill of Benadryl. For people who experience these more severe symptoms, it is important for them to be instructed by their physician in the use of a "bee sting" kit which can be purchased at most pharmacies. The kit contains Benadryl capsules as well as a syringe containing epinephrine which a person should learn to administer.

Some physicians recommend "desensitization" with bee sting venom for those patients who have had a "systemic" reaction in the past. These injections will decrease the severity of the reactions, but there is controversy regarding the long term cost and whether or not they provide protection against anaphylaxis (death) from a sting.

Of the 40 deaths a year from bee stings, almost all occur in the elderly. There is usually no relationship to previous severe reactions and the one that results in death. It is thought that the fatal outcome has as much to do with the arteriosclerosis of the individual as to the sting itself. The child at the ranch who almost died was six years old and had had asthma in the past. On returning from a hike, he complained to his mother of trouble breathing and then suddenly collapsed. His father, a doctor, started mouth to mouth resuscitation. I was called to their cabin immediately and assisted in CPR. The child recovered and was soon his normal self again. The outcome would certainly have been different if no one had known CPR—another excellent reason for EVERYONE to learn it.

One more reaction to bee stings which I almost forgot—injured pride. While horseback riding, a bee stung one of the horses. The teenage rider was bucked off but escaped injury except for—you guessed it—injured pride.

HEAD INJURY: BRUISING THE BOWL OF JELLO

"Jack and Jill went up the hill to fetch a pail of water, Jack fell down and broke his crown, and Jill came tumbling after." Jill probably got up, brushed herself off and went home. Jack was not so lucky. A head injury (the broken crown) can be very serious and result in permanent damage or death. Jack had to be rushed to the emergency room.

When I assist in brain surgery, I am always amazed at the fragility of the human brain. It has the consistency of thick Jello and yet withstands a great deal of abuse during one's lifetime. Fortunately, after millions of years, the skull has developed into a thick but light shield to protect this most important organ of our body, and it does a remarkable job.

Head injuries come in all degrees of severity. Everyone has hit his/her head at one time and has "seen stars," developed a lump on the scalp and experienced a headache for several hours. This is the mildest form of a concussion, a bruise to the brain. A more severe concussion will produce unconsciousness, lasting from a few minutes to a lifetime.

A mild bruise of the arm or leg may result in only slight swelling of the skin, but a severe bruise will produce marked swelling, bleeding and permanent damage. It is the same with the brain, but the results are more devastating. A bruise of the arm does not heal overnight but will take days, weeks or months, so it is with a bruise of the brain.

What are the after effects of a concussion? Following a moderate concussion with a short period of unconsciousness, there usually will be headaches lasting several days to weeks or months. The greatest concern, however, is for patients who have been unconscious for days, weeks or months. Will they ever wake up and will there be any permanent loss of mental capacity? Each injury is different, but the greater the amount of bleeding within the brain the less the chance for recovery. Age is also a factor; the patient over the age of thirty does not do as well as the one under thirty.

Even with these guidelines, however, doctors admit that at times they are surprised. Patients who have been unconscious for months have recovered slowly and have returned to productive lives. With longer periods of coma there are usually permanent handicaps—but the severity of these vary among patients.

The treatment of head injuries on Maui has taken three giant steps forward the last several years. First was the arrival of Dr. Loren Direnfeld, an outstanding neurologist. Second was the installation of the CT (CAT) scanner at Maui Memorial Hospital. The scanner allows doctors to diagnose intracranial (brain) blood clots. Finally, Dr. Slater, a neurosurgeon, established his practice on Maui. With his arrival, complete care of patients with head injuries became available.

Despite all this advanced care, the best treatment is still prevention. Drive carefully. Don't drink and drive. Use your seat belt. Take care of that bowl of Jello on top of your shoulders. It allows you to think, to love and to enjoy the world around you.

VIETNAM: A WAR TO REMEMBER

I cried as I stood before the Vietnam Wall and read the row upon row of names of the young men and women who lost their lives in that far off little country. The Wall is a powerful statement to all who stand before it. A week later I took my family to see the movie "Platoon," and we witnessed the terrible deaths suffered by the men and women whose names are inscribed on The Wall. May our sons and daughters be safe from the ravages of war.

Last night I was reminded of my own Vietnam experiences as I watched a rerun of "MASH," the adventures of doctors and nurses in an Army hospital during the Korean conflict.

In February 1966, I was given command of the 17th Field Hospital, which was a "VIP" hospital in downtown Saigon. We were responsible for the medical care of the American officers and enlisted men in the different military headquarters within the city. During the next ten months most of our "battlefield experiences" were what you would see any Saturday night in the emergency room of a large city hospital. However, twice during that period of time the Viet Cong blew up BOQ's (bachelor officers' quarters), and we were faced with true mass casualties—fifty at one time and a hundred the next.

My real "MASH" experience was during the last two months of my tour in Vietnam. The new commanding officer of the 17th Field Hospital arrived early, so I was utilized as a surgeon at the 93rd Evac Hospital in Long Binh.

It was truly a "MASH" experience—living in dusty, dirty green tents like the "swamp," partying at night, and trying to forget what life during wartime was all about. The operating rooms were in long quonset huts and the helipad was located just outside. Radar's "sensing" of an incoming helicopter brings back many of those memories.

One of the "justifications" of war is that many new medical advancements are achieved with each conflict. My reply to that would be in several four letter words, for I have seen the results of man trying to destroy man. I lost count of the number of leg amputations I performed on the young men who had the misfortune to step on a mine. There were eyes that will never see again because of the shrapnel. The lacerated livers, ruptured spleens, and perforated intestines from gunshot wounds ceased to be "exciting surgical cases" after the first dozen or so. Fifty-eight thousand of our finest young men and women lost their lives in Vietnam and hundreds of thousands were physically and mentally injured. Some of those young people were from Maui.

I hope that the "MASH" series and movies such as "Platoon" play for generations to come so that young people will learn about the horrors of war, and that the older ones, who make the political decisions to go to war, will never forget that there is no glory in man killing man.

FRACTURED RIB

Tickle a rib if you must, but be careful not to break it. Presently I have two patients in the hospital recovering from the complications of broken ribs, and I'm sure they would like to share their problems with you if they could.

The ribs serve as a protective shield around the lungs and because they are thin and curved, they can bend outward as the lung expands when we breathe. As we grow older and pass the sixty-year mark, the ribs may become brittle. In fact, they have been known to break when Dad gives Mom an affectionate bear hug.

Most fractured or broken ribs occur during an accident, and automobile accidents lead the list. This list is long and includes falls from trees, buildings, and horses, Saturday night brawls, and even slipping and falling against the bathtub at home.

Individuals immediately know that they have hurt themselves. First of all, there is considerable pain over the site of the injury. To add to that, each breath becomes more painful, and the patient wants desperately to find his or her doctor (who is probably out playing golf).

Simple fractured ribs, which do not have a sharp point at the break site, will not require hospitalization and can be treated with pain medication and a rib belt. Patients always object to the term "simple," especially since to them the pain is very "major."

If there is a sharp point of rib at the fracture site, then complications can occur. The point can puncture the lung and cause bleeding or collapsing of the lung. A minor operation must then be performed. The physician will anesthetize the skin and put a small tube into the chest in order to remove the blood and air. This will expand the lung. Rarely is it necessary to do a major operation on the lung for the complications of fractured ribs.

I wish that there were quicker methods of healing the rib, relieving the pain and returning the patient to normal life—but there are not. Several weeks of discomfort are to be expected as nature takes its course in the healing process. While the healing occurs, the patient develops new attitudes. An affectionate hug becomes an act of aggression. A friend who tells a joke to cause laughter is a sadist. And a sneeze is the highest form of self-torture. Be "patient," however; after several weeks you will once again enjoy someone "tickling your rib."

7 Medical Practice

CONTROLLING MEDICAL COSTS

When the bills arrive from the doctor or the hospital, two aspirin may not be enough to treat the headache! The amount of money spent nationally on medical care now consumes 10% of our Gross National Product. Twenty percent of the money spent on medical care is for the doctors' fees, while another 40% goes for hospital bills, and the last 40% for drugs, nursing homes and other expenses. Physicians are often blamed for the cost of the last 80%, but this is like blaming the fireman for the cost of water needed to put out a fire.

Whoever, or whatever, is to blame for these spiralling costs (or even if there is any "blame") may never be determined, but what must be done *now* is to make every effort to keep medical costs affordable.

The consuming public must take a leading role in controlling health costs. To keep costs down they must demand less from the medical profession by taking better care of their own health. Here are some specific suggestions to help you minimize health costs. Avoid going to the doctor's office for minor colds and ailments. Use the many informative and helpful books available on "home health care." Do not frequent the emergency room at night because it is "convenient," especially when a condition can safely be treated the next day by your doctor.

Stop smoking! You did not want to hear that, did you? We could reduce medical costs 25% by eliminating illnesses directly related to smoking. Equally important, do not drink and drive! We already are seeing a decline in accident victims coming into the emergency room because of the tougher "drunk driving" laws and the effective police DUI teams.

Following an operation, when your doctor has determined it is time for you to be discharged, do not ask to stay an additional day just because "It isn't convenient to go home today." A single extra hospital day multiplied by 365 times during the year amounts to ONE HUNDRED THOUSAND DOLLARS in unnecessary hospital costs.

When you hear about someone receiving a million dollar malpractice award for "pain and suffering," you, the consumer, and patients will face higher medical costs because physicians need to meet ever-increasing malpractice insurance fees.

Nursing homes are over crowded with parents and grandparents who used to be cared for at home. Now they are an expense of the government. With life expectancy increasing, this cost will continue to climb.

The future is already here and has brought its medical price tag with it. Coronary bypass surgery, kidney dialysis, and kidney, heart and liver transplants are extremely expensive, but who among you would deny one of these operations to a member of your family if it were necessary?

Americans have the highest standard of medical care in the world, and it will continue to improve. There is no such thing as "cheap but good" medicine, and even though doctors do everything economically possible to control health costs, they need your cooperation. TAKE CARE OF YOUR HEALTH. IT'S A GOOD LONG-TERM INVESTMENT.

FIBERSCOPES –
LOOKING INTO THE BODY

"You're going to put that hose where? My stomach? You must be kidding! It's not going to hurt?"

In the last fifteen years there has been a revolution in the diagnosis of different diseases in medicine by the use of instruments we call flexible fiberoptic "scopes."

Prior to that time, if doctors wished to look into the stomach or into the colon, it was necessary to look through "rigid" metal tubes. These were painful and dangerous to the patient, and perforations or tears of the tissue could occur from these rigid instruments.

Within recent years, inventors discovered that if thousands of glass threads were woven into a "fiberoptic" bundle, the image entering through one end of the bundle of fibers could be visualized at the other end, even if the bundle was tied into a knot.

So a medical inventor put two of these bundles into a flexible or bendable hose about the size of your little finger. With this instrument, light could be sent from one end of the hose to the other. By using a lens, a picture could be sent from the far end back to the person looking at the other end of the hose. Thus was born the fiberoptic "scope."

The original scopes have been improved by modern electronics. A "video-chip" is placed at the far end of the scope and the picture is picked up by the camera chip and passed up the scope electronically. The picture is then visualized on a TV monitor and can be "saved" on a video-cassette.

What physicians had to do was to find an opening into which to insert the scope. The first opening to be transgressed by this instrument was the mouth. The fiberoptic "gastroscope" was passed through the mouth, down the esophagus and into the stomach. As a result the treatment of ulcers and other diseases of the stomach improved immensely. Prior to the use of the fiberoptic gastroscope, doctors relied mainly upon x-rays of the stomach for diagnosis; however, they missed many small lesions and never considered other diagnoses. With the fiberoptic gastroscope, doctors are now able to look directly at ulcers, take biopsies, and even stop the bleeding from some ulcers without resorting to surgery.

The next body opening to be examined was the rectum. A long colonoscope was developed which is about five feet long. That's right—FIVE FEET LONG! With this instrument the entire length of the colon can be examined and biopsies or minor operations performed. The American public learned a great deal about the colonoscope when President Reagan underwent colon cancer diagnosis and surgery.

Prior to the use of the colonoscope, if a patient had a polyp of the colon, he would have required a major abdominal operation. This necessitated a week or two in the hospital, a month off from work, possible complications from the operation and several thousand dollars in medical and hospital expenses.

Now, with the use of the colonoscope, the polyp can be removed in a surgicenter or outpatient clinic and the patient can usually return to work the following day with a very small risk of complications from this procedure. The cost of the polypectomy is only a fraction of the cost of a major operation and hospitalization.

Peritonoscopy is another use of fiberoptic scopes. Through a small incision below the umbilicus (belly button), the scope can be introduced and the abdomen distended with carbon dioxide. The gynecologist can then examine the uterus, ovaries or other pelvic areas. Biopsies can be taken or transection of the fallopian tubes can be performed for sterilization. With the use of the peritoneal scope, the liver also can be examined and biopsies taken if necessary.

Even the orthopedic surgeons were not to be left out of the advances of fiberoptic scopes. They use scopes for operations on torn cartilage in the knee. Knee operations use to require an incision four to six inches long. Now a small 1 inch incision is made, the scope introduced, cartilage visualized and the part that is torn is sniped away to prevent locking of the knee.

My grandfather, who practiced medicine in 1910, would be amazed at the instruments we use today. Likewise, some of today's surgical instruments will be outdated and "old-fashioned" by the year 2000. I can hardly wait to see what the future holds.

THE AMA IS UN-AMERICAN

The American Medical Association's vote to press for a federal law outlawing tobacco advertising and promotion certainly seems "un-American" to me. Since "The American Way" is for organizations to promote more business for its members, the AMA is failing in its obligation. It is estimated that 50% of all cancers are directly related to smoking cigarettes and that 15-25% of visits to doctors' offices are from illnesses due to smoking. It is "un-American" for doctors to try to put themselves out of business.

But that has been medicine's way for the last 100 years. It started with tuberculosis (TB). Medicine was so successful at finding a cure that hundreds of TB sanatoriums had to close for lack of patients. Then it was diphtheria and whooping cough— rarely seen now. Millions of lives were saved, yet pediatricians lost all those patients!!

Smallpox, malaria and plague, historically big killers, have been tamed. In fact, doctors and the health organizations of the world have eliminated smallpox from the face of the earth!

And polio! I remember as a child the fear of drinking from a public fountain. I would end up in the iron lung for sure! Hospitals were filled with children and young adults suffering from polio. Orthopedic surgeons operated on thousands every year to correct the deformities left by this disease. Then Dr. Jonas Salk discovered polio vaccine and lost us all that business. Un-American!

And medicine is still at it. The other night I saw a TV ad paid for by the Emergency Physicians Association. It showed the dangers of drinking and driving—the ER docs sure lost business with that ad! Doctors instruct their patients how to follow better diets and exercise more regularly in order to decrease their risks of heart attacks—bad business practices. Hundreds of millions of dollars are spent each year in medical research, not to find more patients, but to find the cure for cancer, AIDS, arteriosclerosis and other diseases. It certainly seems that medicine is trying to put itself out of business.

Think what would happen if other businesses followed medicine's example. Airlines would advertise for you to stay home and enjoy your savings. McDonald's would teach home cooking. Nissan would tell you how to make your old Datsun run like new for another five years. And lawyers would use their TV ads to encourage you to shake hands and solve your problems on a friendly basis. All "un-American!"

Medicine may be the most "un-American" of all the businesses, but it is the greatest of all professions. I am proud to be one of its members.

Index